THE POWER OF HUMAN ENERGY

How to Raise Your Positive Energy and Use it to Achieve a Fulfilled and Happy Life

Guide, Techniques, Meditations and Exercises

RENATA FRANCETIĆ

Author: Renata Francetić
Title: The Power of Human Energy
Subtitle:
How to Raise Your Positive Energy and Use it to Achieve a Fulfilled and Happy Life
Guide, Techniques, Meditations and Exercises

Publisher: Author's Own Edition
Place and Year of Issue: Zagreb, 2020.
Type of Publication: Spirituality and Religion
URL: www.glossyenergy.blog
E-mail: glossyenergy@gmail.com

ISBN 978-953-49111-0-5
A CIP catalog record of this book is available from the National and University Library in Zagreb under number 001069185.

Contents

Introduction

I have long been preparing and adding to this book in my mind over the past twenty-five years. Sooner or later, we all become aware, to a greater or lesser extent, that the manner in which we have been brought up; the manner in which they tried to force us to behave; the manner in which the media and people around us, even now, wish to influence us, the way we think, and the way we act are not the things that determine who we are as people. We are somebody else.

It is very difficult to be different in a world that is constantly trying to mold us according to itself. Few people have the strength to resist this influence and choose their own path. Generally, under these kinds of circumstances the only person you can rely on is yourself. At that point you come to the understanding, as I did, that the only way to stand up to everything and everyone is with faith in God. When I began in my twenties to resist all external negative elements, they thought that I wouldn't be able to adapt to the world; if you were different, you would be judged and rejected. I asked myself what this meant to them. From a young age, I knew what was right and what was not. I always behaved according to fairness and the truth. Today's world ignores this, rejects it, and mocks it. Because of this, today's world and today's society are falling into ever deeper chaos, there is ever greater alienation in families, and the family has, like society, lost its value, strength and power.

No matter how much they tried to convince me that this kind of path of fairness and truth was impossible in today's world, I always kept to it, accompanied by the immeasurable strength of my faith in God. I am still keeping to it today, and that is how it will remain. I have never taken the path of least resistance, and I have always known that I am living in the right way.

Due to my great faith in God, I began to feel His presence and His support. Now, after 25 years of my difficult path through life, with God's help, things happen simply and are resolved simply. The things that for others are resolved with a great deal of struggle and upset happen to me in exactly the way that is best for me. I am always calm and I always find a positive message because I look at everything as another life lesson. God taught me that every effect has its cause. If I treat others with respect, understanding, and honesty, the positive energy that I project towards them in that moment cannot allow them to behave towards me in any unacceptable way.

From my own experience, I know that with an increase of positive energy, which means a vast understanding of myself, my approaches, and the situations I find myself in, as well as an openness in the way I look at the people I meet, I must approach every situation in life with a mind that is wide open. When I look at my beginnings and current situation, I know that it was harder to accept my role of an open heart towards God and behavior in keeping with His teachings, a life lived in love for Him, myself and the people around me, rather than all the words, contempt and bad behavior of the people who tried, in various ways, to lead me away from my path and who mocked my way of life.

I can always tell you that this path paid off, that I am now in a situation where I always know the answer to all the situations that occur to me in my life, that I always know how to help a person in the way that they need most. I can sympathize, I can understand, I know how to give advice, and I know when I need to stay silent and not act.

Thanks to my deep connection with God, in the past few years of my life, things have happened that have made my life easier. I have been given ideas and problems have resolved themselves. I am following the course that God leads me on thanks to the openness of my mind and the development of my consciousness. Nothing can surprise me anymore; nothing can disappoint me or hurt me. I know I am protected.

It is incredibly difficult to begin and persevere on this difficult path. People usually give up. I can only advise you to persevere, and it will pay off.

I wrote this book as an aid to those who want to change the way they live their lives but don't know how. This is a difficult path, but it is the only satisfactory and valuable one, and one that we will all have to follow sooner or later. Nobody can avoid learning who they are at their core. We all want to be loved and supported as we are.

So be positive, think positively, behave positively, do positive things, and this will lead you to the path of enlightenment that every person longs for consciously and unconsciously. This is the path that leads to love, joy, luck, and good health.

PART I

The Human Body

All that was created came out of the energy of Love, the all-Pervasive energy of all that is visible and invisible, all that is created and uncreated, all that is animate and inanimate.

The human body consists of five parts that form a unified whole. These parts are the physical, psychic, mental, spiritual, and the soul. Each of these five bodies has its own energy body without which the human body cannot function. Furthermore, every human body has nine energy centers. Seven energy centers are related to the first three parts (the physical, psychic, and mental), and two energy centers are related to the spiritual and the soul.

The physical body consists of the digestive systems, the motor system, the nervous system, and the bones, which in the human body are only fully developed once an individual reaches twenty-one years of age.

The psychic body refers to emotions we accept during our lifetime.

The mental body refers to thoughts, which do not cease from the time of our birth until our physical death.

The soul is the energy that is received when our physical body is conceived, and it remains in our physical body until the death of the physical body, after which it returns back to its Source and is never completely lost.

The spiritual body is the energy that is eternally connected to our Source.

The human body was made perfect. Its proper use, the consumption of high-quality food, high-quality energy, and correct, positive thoughts enable it to have a healthy life and helps in realizing the reasons for your having entered into a physical body at precisely this moment, in this place, with these people, in this environment and these circumstances. Everything that happens within you and around you are here for a reason. You have chosen what to experience in this life; therefore, people, environments, and events were given to you so that you might realize the reason for your arrival on Earth.

The seven energy centers that are related to the first three human bodies are absolutely interconnected and intertwined. The first center refers to the regulation of balance and it includes the legs. The second center refers to the reproductive organs, kidneys, bladder, bowels, and their interconnections. The third center is the solar plexus, as well as the stomach, spleen, pancreas, gallbladder, and their interconnections. The fourth center is the heart area, which encompasses the heart, lungs, bronchia, and their interconnections, as well as the arms. The fifth center encompasses the thyroid gland and the four epithelial bodies, as well as the throat and neck. The sixth center includes the third eye (the pineal gland), sinuses, teeth, and their interconnections. The seventh center is the brain.

The two energy centers that are related to the spiritual body and the soul are situated in two locations within the body. When a person is standing straight or sitting with a straight spine, he or she is connected to the Earth's energy and the energy of the Universe. These two centers are the most active at the time. The center connected to the Earth is about four centimeters below the belly button in the middle of that part of the body, while the center connected to the Universe is about twelve centimeters below the last neckline in the heart energy area, in the middle of that part of the body.

When all nine energy centers are connected, the body is then in absolute balance with itself, with the Earth's energy and the energy of the Universe; in other words, it is absolutely healthy.

Each of the seven energy centers has its own color. The first center is red, the second orange, the third yellow, the fourth green, the fifth blue, the sixth indigo (violet-blue), and the seventh is golden or white.

Because the human body is pure energy – both positive and negative – each cell has its own polarity. Each cell is, on the one hand, positive and, on the other hand, negative. This is the reason why all cells mutually attract or repulse one another. Every human body has a frequency at which it functions, and this frequency is completely different from the frequencies of other people.

Every organ, gland, and all parts of the physical body have their own precisely defined cell structure, which means that the cells of every body part are completely different. Each cell contains an awareness that enables it to regenerate in the same way it was created. If cells are exposed to negative energies, cell mutation occurs. Firstly, cell mutation is observed in the energy field of our mental body, then in our psychic body, and afterwards in our physical body. Consequently, an illness appears.

All cells in the body are renewed approximately every eleven months.

Every organ reacts to your thoughts on it. If you do not treat one of your organs with respect, it reacts to your negative energy, and pain appears. This warns you that your way of thinking does not suit it, nor you as a whole organism. For example, when a woman has strong menstrual discharge and does not treat her uterus with respect, she begins to feel pain during her menstrual cycles. The angrier and more furious she gets, the more she will begin to feel greater problems over time. Later, the problems occur even several days prior to and after the cycle.

Accept your organs with love because they will not be able to provide you with what they are here to provide, which is to ensure the perfect and healthy functioning of your physical body.

Your body has been given to you to use so that you can fulfill the purpose of your reincarnation, so it is necessary to treat it with love and respect.

The body is able to heal itself because it is made up of the positive energy that you received when you were born. If you believe in this, it shall be so. You yourself are familiar with numerous examples showing that, when you would cut or injure yourself, the body healed itself, or when there was a bone fracture, a bone that was set healed itself. Respect your body and love it, and it will serve you for a long time.

Food for the Physical Body

Food for the physical body is the food we eat, as well as water.

Every plant grown naturally, or plants from areas where they grow on their own, has a high energy and is therefore a high-quality source of nourishment. All plants grow in a particular part of the year. In the period when it ripens naturally, its fruit is of the greatest quality; in other words, it contains the most high-quality energy for the human body. People should eat plants whose habitat is the territory where they themselves reside. This means that a certain group of people is compatible with food that grows where they are stationed; such food suits them best energy-wise. Food invented by the human mind, such as snacks, sweets, and fast food, is not suitable for the human body because it contains a low level of energy, if any. The consumption of such food, especially in younger people (up to twelve years of age) leads to cell mutation and unwanted consequences later in life. Nowadays, corpulence (obesity) is very common. Being obese differs from being fat because fat occurs as a consequence of the incorrect consumption of food that is derived from nature by people, which refers to fruit, vegetables, meat and fish.

Everything that enters the body should be consumed with respect, because in that way, you are telling your body that you love and respect it. Everybody has its own rhythm, which means that everything is defined during birth. There are night and day; times when the human body is more or less active. Night was created in order for the physical body to rest from its daily activities, food, and events. Since your thoughts are constantly at work, night is the time when your body analyzes the previous day, sometimes other and even longer periods, and tries to understand or find a way out of a certain situation, if necessary. If one does not sleep during the period created for sleeping, the whole body becomes dysfunctional and a person can have issues with insomnia, digestion, and nerves. This means that in twenty-four hours, a person needs approximately 5 to 7 hours of sleep at nighttime. In some situations, due to some people's working hours, it is not possible, but this is rare.

Water is a component that makes up approximately seventy-five percent of the human body. The water we ingest should be the water that "falls from the skies," or rainwater. Such water is free from the negative energy that is accumulating in the Earth today, which is present in bottled water. Tap water in cities is also polluted, so it is better not to drink it, nor use it for food preparation, if possible.

For people who drink tap water, because taps are made out of metal and therefore release a part of that metal every time a tap is opened, this metal accumulates in the body. Given the fact that our body does not need this kind of metal, especially not metal obtained in such a way, the body tries to free itself from such metals either through absorption or disposal. The constant intake of such water prevents the organism from performing the same function over and over because it is becoming tired, and the body begins sending you signal that this does not suit it. It is your task to listen to it. Should you fail to listen to it, illnesses will develop, which are reflected in your physical body.

Pure water is highly energized, full of beautiful crystals, the shapes that can be seen in snowflakes. Studies were conducted on water, polluted water, water exposed to positive words (love, respect, satisfaction), water exposed to negative words (fear, rage, disease), water exposed to noise, water exposed to classical music, and others. Polluted water was affected by deep prayer and love-filled meditation. After some time, it was purified completely, and it was filled with beautiful crystals.

Since water contains energy, the water reacted to everything that contained positive energy in a positive manner, and it created crystals, while it reacted to negative energy by becoming murky and the beautiful crystals did not appear. The human body reacts in the same way.

Water is a healthy fluid because it improves digestion, and in some cases, calms the body, but water should not be over-ingested because too much water increases the pressure on the kidneys and makes them weak. Today's water, if not filtered, contains a lot of chlorine and limescale, which are detrimental for the body. There is a chance that kidney stones will develop.

A person who lives only off plants (vegetables, fruit, cereals, and mushrooms) ingests the fluid and energy of those plants. For such people it is enough to ingest about one liter of fluids, including juice, soup, vegetables, fruit, cereal preparations, and water. During the summer, due to perspiration, it is necessary to drink up to one liter of fluid more than usual.

People who eat heavy foods, such as animal meat and fish, need more fluids for easier digestion. Such people need up to four liters of fluid daily. During the summer, due to perspiration, it is necessary to ingest up to one and a half liters of fluid more than usual.

Since everything you ingest contains energy, some food combinations cancel out each other's energies, so when ingesting food, it might happen that the food does not perform its function, or in other words, it does not give you the necessary energy, and you then feel tired. The consumption of vegetables makes you feel light, while the consumption of animal meat and fish can make you feel heavy. One of the biggest mistakes is to consume various types of food all at once. The best thing to do is to eat one type of food, then wait for about ten minutes for the stomach to finish its work, and then ingest another type of food until everything is eaten. When consuming plants, you can eat everything together.

Given the various energies of particular foods, it is not good to mix meat and potatoes because after that, a person feels a great weight. Furthermore, it is not good to use onion and garlic together while preparing food because they are energetically opposites and lose their healing properties.

The goal of most foods that are prepared these days is to please our palate, and we do not think about their healing properties for our physical body, which is inescapable.

Some people who consider themselves vegetarians, by which one I refer to people who eat neither meat nor fish, nor animal products such as milk and eggs, think that their children (small children) should follow the same diet. Most cereals are inappropriate for children until the age of seven because they are energetically extremely strong in contrast to a child's subtle and gentle energy, and in using them, children are harmed, not benefited. By this, I am referring primarily to soymilk. For children, cow's milk is appropriate, as well as a lot of fruit and vegetables, with the smallest possible amount of sugar. They get enough sugar from fruit. If a child refuses to eat a particular type of fruit or vegetable, do not force them if it is not necessary, but at the same time, do not give them replacement foods in the sense of sweets and other types of foods containing sugar simply so they eat something. Children should not consume mushrooms before the age of ten because their stomachs are not developed enough to digest them.

If the body is healthy, a small amount of salt is necessary, especially during the summer, when salt is excreted through perspiration.

The same applies to everything you ingest; your body always reacts. Rest for about thirty minutes after every meal so that your stomach can do it's work. If you feel light and full after that, such food suits you. The stomach should never be completely full. It is better to eat smaller meals four times per day. When you put food in your mouth, chew it because the teeth and saliva, which has antibacterial properties, must do their work, and only afterwards should you swallow. When eating solid food do not consume water or other fluids, because you should allow the stomach to do its work. After eating, you may drink something only after thirty minutes.

Every cooked meal should be set aside for a while to cool to body temperature. Only then is it in the best state for your physical body. In addition, warm meals must only be eaten within three hours of preparation; after three hours they lose their energetic properties. Some types of food must not be eaten when cool because they are harmful (toxic) for your body. These include, for instance, cold spinach or baked potatoes.

Every body is different and has a different energy, so it should be treated as unique. Some bodies are suited for ingesting more vegetables, some more fruit, as well as animal products and related foods, such as milk, eggs, and cheese. Not a single body is fit for ingesting animal meat, whether it be from animals that walk, fly, or swim. The majority of animals consumed by humans have suffered certain negative experiences: choking, slaughtering, or suffocation. Such negative energies remain within the animals' bodies, and humans, by consuming such meat, absorb all of these energies into their bodies, where they remain.

Because almost nobody prays deeply with comprehension, prayer is necessary prior to the consumption of food. Most people pray by saying "God, bless the food we are about to eat to replenish our bodies or my body". This is a prayer that in most cases does not carry great strength or even any because it is said as an obligation or a necessity. Correct prayer would thank the animal that gave its life for your meal and ask for forgiveness for all that it went through to reach your table.

The human body is made in such a way that it does not need to consume the flesh of either animals or fish. It is widely known that people who consume animal meat in small amounts or not at all are healthier than those who do so. In the Holy Bible, the first page tells us: "Let us make human beings in our image, after our likeness. Let them have dominion over the fish of the sea, the birds of the air, the tame animals, all the wild animals, and all the creatures that crawl on the earth."

Having dominion means taking care of them, not destroying them, multiplying them by force, killing them, or crossing species. Such behavior is detrimental for both the human species and animals, as well as for plants. In addition, it mentions the kind of food that was meant for humans: "See, I give you every seed-bearing plant on all the earth and every tree that has seed-bearing fruit on it to be your food!"

Animals have a different frequency, lower than that of humans. They are therefore not suitable for consumption. Such food harms the body by reducing its energy. Plants often have pure energy because it is received directly from Mother Earth and the Sun.

Food represents sustenance and purification for the physical body for it to increase its life energy. Food is ingested for the energy it gives to the body, not because, as some see it, of the amount needed to make the physical body function. The food that people consume is primarily here for the energy it gives to the physical body, not the amount of vitamins and minerals it contains.

God made the human body perfect. By providing it with food that has a large amount of positive energy, while not being too heavy for the body, you enable it to be what it was made to be. The body is created so that each organ and each gland produces with a healthy lifestyle and nutrition the amount of vitamins and minerals necessary for that particular body. Each body is different, so everyone should listen to their bodies to provide them with foods that are acceptable for the type of body they have. Everything that appeals to the palate – and such foods are numerous – is, for the most part, bad for your body because it lowers your energy.

It is widely known that Tibetan hermits only eat *tsampa* (coarsely ground wheat flour) and rainwater, and some live up to four hundred years. The amount of food ingested or its variety is irrelevant; the quality of the food in terms of its energy is important.

The reason why we have entered into a physical body is to increase our body's energy, which means that our body's energy becomes pure and light. Such energy is possessed by the Saints. It is clear that anybody can be a saint. It is all a matter of making the decision and possessing the desire to achieve purification.

Food for the Psychic Body

Every body reacts to exposure to the positive and negative energies of emotions.

When a body feels positive energy, including the strongest energy of love, it is exhilarated, it functions perfectly. People feel healthy, free, without pressure, without stress, and without any problems; they emanate positive energy. Other people experience the desire to be close to those kinds of people because they inspire the people around them, bringing a peace and joy that radiates from them. All other positive emotions affect a person in the same way: positively and in a manner that heals the body and creates joy, happiness, satisfaction, attention, kindness, peace, friendship, giving, tenderness, and other emotions that make you feel good and exalted in your own body.

Benevolence is one of the greatest virtues. Every time a person does a good deed and does not expect anything in return, they feel good in their own bodies. Their energy increases because they have felt one type of endless and unconditional love and in that way, their energy increases and the body heals itself. If you feel any negative energy related to the good deeds you have done and expect something in return from that person, you decrease your energy and close off your heart. The body is then suffocated, and illness occurs in the physical body, mostly in the areas of the thyroid gland, the heart, or the solar plexus.

Satisfaction is a feeling you do not need to share with anybody except yourself. If you think that the people you would like to share your satisfaction with would not react in a suitable way and support you, then keep your satisfaction to yourself and enjoy it. If you know that people who are extremely important to you would not react positively and supportively to your feeling of satisfaction, then you should know that they are not ready to share positive things with you. There is a time for everything; do not rush ahead. Sometimes that time comes when you find yourself on the same wavelength with such people and you can tell them about your satisfaction in order to share it and mutually increase your positive energies. But sometimes this does not happen. You should not feel sorry about this. If you are on the path towards healing your body and someone else is not ready for it right now, do not worry; when the time comes, they will be. Nobody has ever stood in one place. Everyone arrives where they should be, in an easier or harder way, indirectly or straight; nobody is lost nor will they ever be.

Peace is the state closest to the body's needs. When the body is at peace, it means that you are not tortured by worries or problems, which is the most important thing for your body's health. It also means that you have correctly understood the words "leave your problems to God". It means that you have understood that every problem has its source or cause and that you need to understand why it appeared. Everything occurs so you can learn something. If you do not understand or recognize your problems, they will recur, very likely in the same – or in a similar – form. They will accumulate because you are not resolving them. They will smother and pressure you, and you will lose your sense of peace. Some people think that they never even had it to begin with. You had it. You will find it again. You just have to choose it, and if you do not find it, it will find you.

The act of giving is something we receive at birth. Giving from the heart without asking for something in return does not cost a thing It brings you satisfaction and joy; it fills your heart, increases your energy, and in doing so, it purifies you. This is why people who give are healthier and happier than those who do not treat in such a way, their nearest and dearest, meaning people they are in contact with, as well as plants, animals, and the Earth. Everyone can give out of love; it is only a question of whether they want to do it, and whether they realize their own wellbeing in doing so.

Friendship is a different feeling from the ones we have mentioned above. In friendship, there is mutual, selfless giving. Many perceive friendship as a state in which they can ask anything from a person and they, if they are true friends, would do it unconditionally and without objection. This is not friendship; this is a superior-subordinate relationship. Such a relationship can be maintained as long as both sides are willing to play those roles. The correct kind of friendship exists only if all people within that close circle – meaning up to four people – are satisfied, calm, and relaxed. With true friendship, people can always find understanding and help that is suitable to the problem that has emerged. Friendships do not suffer fights or conflicts, and regardless of separation, friendship is unwavering.

Paying attention refers to accepting the situations that occur to you with understanding. Most people walk through life uncontrollably, which means that they do not notice anything, whether it be a situation that is related to them or to their immediate or distant surroundings. Most people do not know what their neighbor looks like or their neighbor's name. They do not know who works in the office next door or why they always go to the same store. They are here and walk the Earth because they think somebody has pushed them and forced them to live this life. It is not so, nor will it ever be, because everything happens to you and around you for a reason. Therefore, open your eyes and enjoy the variety of life. This world is full of colors, smells, and tastes; pay attention to it and live.

Tenderness is the feeling that fills our hearts the most. It can be communicated through a touch, a voice, a look. Give tenderness to everything in your surroundings. Each being is at its core tender, so jeopardizing this feeling, with any negative energy, leaves a deep mark.

Infatuation is felt by everyone at least once in a lifetime. Infatuation must not be mistaken for love. Infatuation occurs because of a certain state of consciousness. It can occur because a person is amorous by nature, because they like something specific on the physical body of another person, because of their personality, or because of a compatibility of energies, which means that their frequencies are on the same level, and so on. The reasons why somebody may fall in love are incredibly numerous. Sometimes infatuation is steady enough that people remain together for the rest of their lives. Usually, it is not. Most people who stay together do not do so out of infatuation but for many different reasons.

Love is energy. Nothing exists outside of it. When you love someone, there is no possibility of falling out of love and falling in love again. It is impossible. Love *is*. There are not many couples on this Earth who can confirm this. Love is unconditional and always equally strong, no matter what. Love that can be called so is mostly love between a mother and her biological child. Other real loves, such as a love between partners, are scarce.

We connect sex to infatuation, which can be very good or very bad, as well as violent (I would not recommend that to anybody because it is very dangerous to play the role of a tyrant/victim and every cause has its effect, which means that roles can swap in order for a person to realize what is wrong with such an attitude). In sex, only physical bodies are connected. In love, there is lovemaking, where, apart from physical bodies, souls connect as well, and it can happen that only souls are connected (and the physical body is completely satisfied in equal measure).

Infatuation is blind. Love is ever-present and fulfilling, and the person experiencing it feels whole. The color of infatuation is red, and it denotes sex, blood, war, and violence, while the color of love is light pink and expresses tenderness and attachment.

Patience is the greatest of virtues. Patience tells your body that it is welcome, that you are listening to it, that you know what it needs, and that you will do anything to satisfy it and make it happy, which leads to good health.

Kindness is a feeling that is often misinterpreted. Most people who are said to be kind actually let others humiliate and use them. Kind people must first be good to themselves. This means that they have to respect, appreciate and love themselves. Such energy is projected onto other people, so they do not consider their kindness, giving and dedication as an act of exploitation but rather pure kindness. When people do not appreciate themselves, they are letting their body know that they are not good enough, that they hate themselves.

Fear is the strongest negative emotion. It creates a total blockage in your body within all its energy centers. It closes off your body's energy and leads to illness. Nowadays fear is present in most people. People ascribe it extreme importance. Since they feed this sense of importance, the fear grows and is extremely strong. People thus believe that it is a natural state of consciousness because of these circumstances and external influences, and that they cannot do anything about this situation, this problem. As long as you ascribe such importance to fear, it will continue to saturate you, to decrease your energy and make you an unhealthy person, filled with wrath, frustration, stress, rage, depression and hate.

Hate is a feeling that creates blockages in parts of the physical body where the body's immunity is weaker, which means that the body cannot fight off various diseases effectively because you have weakened it with numerous negative thoughts.

Revenge is a diseased state because a person who has been hurt does not understand why such a thing has happened, and with the existing negative energy that comes from having been hurt, that person feels less valuable and feels an even heavier negative energy, the desire for revenge. Revenge corrodes the body and leads to serious illnesses in the abdominal part (the stomach) of the body.

Rage is an extremely negative emotion that leads to severe diseases such as cancer and tumors. Similarly, problems with weight can occur, because when you express rage towards your body it realizes that you do not want it or need it and that you want to get rid of it.

Anger can lead to Alzheimer's disease. Most people get angry when they do not get their way. Many have a prominent ego, and anger is their way of communicating in order to get what their ego needs, regardless of whether they, or the people around them, are okay with it or not. Such people do not see anybody but themselves. You will feel that they are watching you closely, but you will be able to see that what you say does not register with them. They are wrapped up in their own thoughts, wishes, and nothing and nobody exists but them. Such people feel lonely and constantly seek the company of people who will compliment them and tell them that they are always right.

Humiliation is a feeling experienced by most people, a feeling that occurs when a person is insecure, which means that they do not feel supported by the people around them. People lacking in energy feel humiliation. Nobody needs to support you apart from yourself. Nobody can have as much love and understanding for you, apart from yourself. Focus on yourself and you will find the truth. The truth liberates you, so you will be free.

Concern show how strong and how deep your faith in God is. People who are distanced from themselves and from God feel concern for all. They enjoy saying that they are concerned about something. They want to draw attention to themselves, to show that they are caring people who need to be appreciated and loved, and since they worry about everything, that they should be listened to because they know best.

Stubbornness is a trait in people who always have to have their own way regardless of whether they are right or not – and they know if they are right or not – whether others like it or not, whether it is useful for them and/or others or not. For them, the principle of the matter is 'I stand behind it'. These are stern people who do not give up on their attitudes, and it is difficult to make them think outside their boundaries.

Insecurity is more common in the young than it is in older people. Most people connect their insecurities with their life experiences, which is wrong. Insecure people are the ones who do not believe in themselves and their possibilities. The majority of older people are in the same situation, but they have learned to hide it, while in younger people, it is visible.

An inability to commit is present in people who were hurt, who are unsure of themselves and the possibility of providing and keeping a person they like, or who think they are not worthy of love and attention.

Helplessness is present in most situations in which a person cannot actively participate but has to adapt and act with respect to the situation, whether they like it or not. All situations should be considered from an outside the observer's point of view, not from that of the participant, and in doing so a person can realize why they need to experience that situation and what they can learn from it.

Depression is isolation, separation from God. Depression is a consequence of ignorance and a lack of the desire to find out the truth about ourselves, who we really are.

Many people are not aware of their negative emotions. Therefore, they cannot understand them or resolve them either. Most people express their negative attitudes and feelings through violence and aggression. They are thus demonstrating that they need the energy of love that permeates all negative energies, leaving nothing but love behind.

In the same way many men, more so than women, run from themselves these days. This running away is expressed in an inability to stay in one place for a longer period of time (for instance, staying in their apartment for three hours) in peace; instead, they constantly have to be on the move. Such people do not want to understand that they have a serious problem, which they must face if they want to feel better. They are usually frustrated, tense, think that they have to do everything by themselves, worry about the smallest trifles. The problems that may occur are sudden jerks, facial stiffness, heart palpitations, insecurity, and anxiety.

All negative emotions are subjective and surreal because they are not the true nature of your state of being. Once a person realizes this, they are liberated and become a being of love, carefree, and happy.

Everything is connected; you create your body based on what you bring into it through your emotions. One without the other does not function. By bringing in positive energy through positive emotions, your body functions in a natural way.

Everything is predetermined by our reincarnation.

People limit themselves with their attitudes and way of thinking. God created us unlimited! Never demean your appearance!

Food for the Mental Body

Your thoughts are food for your mental body. From the moment you are born, up until your physical death, your brain is constantly at work. Therefore, it is necessary to control your thoughts.

Your thoughts are constantly creating a mental picture of your wishes. Mental thoughts that are stronger and more defined usually develop into a strong wish or need, which means that they move up to the next level, the psychological level of your body. If you still have a strong wish to make the image in your mind a reality, it will be reflected on the physical level, it will materialize. That is how the commonly discussed process works – thought, word and deed.

Given that you define and determine what you are with your thoughts, or what you want to be, it is necessary to control them and direct them in a certain way.

In children up to the age of twelve, thoughts are mostly directed towards play, food, and their guardians, as well as their immediate environment. A young person older than twelve years of age starts developing their own way of thinking and defining of their thoughts. From age twelve until age twenty-five, our thoughts are chaotic. Therefore, most young people seek noise in order to silence the storm of their thoughts. Noise and loud music are incredibly harmful for your body because they make it nervous and restless, and besides that, permanently damage your hearing. This mode of expression makes the already difficult task of growing up and accepting oneself even harder. To get rid of chaotic thoughts, it is simpler to engage in meditation or sports. It can be an individual sport for which you do not need another person, such as roller-skating or riding a bike. If you are more inclined towards team sports, choose to engage in them. In engaging in anything you are interested in, you will not only calm your chaotic thoughts, but also create a balance in your body.

Young people who have any health issues whatsoever can freely engage in meditation and always pray to their higher “self”, their higher consciousness, God, for guidance.

After the age of twenty-five, people should direct their efforts towards controlling their own thoughts. In other words, they should define what they want in life and in the near future, and what kind of a person they want to be. By defining your needs, you lead your thoughts in the right direction. Great determination is necessary in order to achieve your goals.

Given that thoughts continuously appear in your head and constantly interchange, to control them it is necessary to direct your attention towards them and become aware of them.

After you become aware of them, you should begin observing them. You will see that they change according to an unusual order and are of different lengths. In their minds, most people focus on retelling events that affected them in a positive or negative way. When you finally understand what these events are, try to understand what those thoughts represent for you. Most people, emotionally, on a psychological level, continuously repeat the same event. This means that they did not understand it. Understanding what happened to you means realizing what happened, why it happened, and what you need to learn from it.

The next step is control over your thoughts. This refers to a situation in which a thought starts running through your mind. You should stop it and tell yourself that it is enough, move on; I have understood you and I do not need you anymore.

Try to relax during this exercise, because then you have greater control over yourself and your thoughts. Real control over your mind is made up of thoughts without thoughts. That means that you let yourself accept limitless positive energy from the omniscient Universe. Then you are a person without cares because you know that everything will resolve itself in the best possible way at a particular moment. This exercise can be done during the day. Sit with your back straight and relax as much as you can. Do not cross your legs or arms. Gaze at a monochromatic and light background, such as a wall. Close your eyes slowly and try to keep that monochromatic picture of a wall in your mind. The longer you practice, the better results you will have.

After you define those thoughts relating to what you want from your life, keep those images in mind. You have to be extremely determined, but always think about whether something like that will help you personally and ensure the growth of your soul. If it is not good for you, and if you or anyone else will learn nothing or receive nothing good from your wish which becoming a reality, your thoughts will not come true.

Everything you do, do it for your own good and the good of others, and success is guaranteed. In this way, you raise your body's energy levels and the energy of your surroundings. By surroundings, we mean people, animals, plants, and the Earth.

When you correctly define a thought you want realized, create an image in your head, and if that is a problem, you can draw it on a piece of paper, or simply write down the wish on a piece of paper and always keep it nearby. You should sometimes look at it or read it. Each time you look at it, you should feel joy and happiness in your body, as if it has already come true, as if you already have it.

Since your thoughts are realized first on a psychological level, it is necessary to deal exclusively with positive thoughts. Your positive thoughts increase your body's positive energy, and in that way, they strengthen your immune system. Therefore, you should always think about yourself in a positive way. The only reason why you are here, in this place, is because of God's desire, and your own desire to learn something and to grow, which means realizing who and what you are. Since it is so, the only thing you need to seek is support from yourself because just by being here, you receive God's support, you always have and always will.

By controlling your thoughts and calming them, you come into direct contact with yourself and you then understand who you truly are. After that, you will always look for support in yourself and you will always have it!

Food for the Spiritual Body and the Soul

Food for the spiritual body and the soul is the positive energy of love, which is an eternal and constant force of positive energy. It has been in your body since you were born and will remain there until the death of your physical body. It has always existed and always will; it is eternal.

PART II

Influence and Shaping of a Person up to twelve Years of Age

People who take care of children from the time that the child is born do not, for the most part, understand what their duty in raising such a young person really is. Children have a fine, subtle energy that is very sensitive to the energy of their environment. It is usually said that it is necessary for a child to be with its mother until the age of three. In addition, it is not acceptable for a child to be exposed to various energies, various people, after it is born and up until it is three months old. Since a child's energy is very susceptible to external energies, a newborn may die if it finds itself in close proximity to a very negative person. When a child is next to its mother, it is protected by her energy of love, which is the reason why most babies are healthy up to the age of three.

The duty of a parent or guardian is to understand the child, its wishes and needs, and to not take their own childhood frustrations out on it. Every human being has come into this world for a particular reason, each has come with a particular purpose that needs to be fulfilled; it is the purpose of life, growth in a spiritual direction, an understanding of the self, acceptance of the self, and the understanding that we are all the same before God, since we were born because of him at this moment and in this place.

By taking out their frustrations on their child, parents or guardians suppress the real need of the child's purpose. Depending on the strength of this suppression, including the character of the young being, it often happens that the majority of such people do not have the will to find out the truth about themselves. Therefore, we can observe that most people nowadays live uncontrollably, without goals or any desire to change. Everybody else is to blame for what is going on in his or her life and for the environment they live in.

Those who are stronger in character must first resist the energy of suppression that grows with age because a parent or a guardian feeds them daily with their energy. In order to understand that, it is necessary to think about oneself, not in the sense of their parents and guardians but as individual beings.

Parents or guardians transfer their energy, which is for the most part negative (imbalanced), onto a younger being through behavior, speech, looks, and touch partially to free themselves of it. In such a way, they lower the young being's energy and the child often falls ill. It mostly manifests as aggressive behavior or psychological problems. When young people visit the doctor, they mostly do not look for the cause of the problem but only observe the illness. It has always been a problem in treatment that doctors rarely look for a cause of disease that originates in the psyche and is mental, and in young people, there is usually a problem in their environment.

Since a child only seeks love, understanding and support, when it does not find it, arrogance appears, as well as seeking, nagging, blackmail, and other things you think a child does out of spite. The only thing it seeks in that moment is attention. By punishing the child for that behavior, you are letting the child know that understanding it is irrelevant, that you are always right, so-called parental or guardian selfishness occurs, and that it shall always be as you say because you are certainly smarter than your child. Your children are often smarter and more intelligent than you. Children inherit only twenty-five percent of their character and physical appearance from their parents; they inherit the rest from their ancestors.

The majority of attitudes that cause frustration and problems in older children are:

- you are not good enough
- how could this happen to you
- what were you thinking
- you don't think
- you are so stupid, everybody knows that
- he/she is better than you
- you have to be the best
- I won't give you..., if you don't do... and...
- do you think I will do your thinking for you your whole life

Among the very worst attitudes is disregard.

They are truly numerous. By behaving in this way, you create frustration in your children that is strongly reflected in their later lives. They keep telling themselves that they are not good enough. Later, the things that are triggered are pain, instability, insecurity, escaping from reality, avoiding the truth, living a lie, fits of rage, arrogance, aggression, and smugness.

I place an emphasis on disregard because people become completely isolated, withdrawn, and convinced that they are not worthy of love.

All this happens because you did not provide your children with what they needed. Every child is a person who carries the energy of the events it experienced in previous incarnations. It brings this along in order to ease the understanding and acceptance of events that will take place over the course of its physical life. It is up to you to follow it, see its affinities and needs, and, with respect to the situation nowadays, direct it in the best possible way, the best way you know how.

Most children are insatiable when asking their parents or guardians questions. You must answer all their questions but adapt your answers to your child's age.

Also, let your child express itself freely and let it tell you everything, always and at each and every moment. Most parents see their child through themselves, which is absolutely wrong since every child, every person, is an individual being. Your child is not you; it is unique in every sense: its behavior, character, and reactions to similar things in life are different. Understand your child's words in the way they are said, not in the way that you would describe them with all your life experience, because you will always be wrong. Children say what they mean, except if they lose trust in you because of your lies, so take every word as it was said.

Since children, up to the age of twelve do not understand your words but feel them, understanding body language and behavior, you cannot cheat them even if you tried. So be careful not only about what you say, but how you say it, and what kind of energy you reflect with your words and attitudes. With such a relationship, you will raise children who will not trust you later in life, who will not ask for advice, or with whom you will not be able to communicate; children will retaliate or lie because they have lost faith in you. You will wonder how it happened and lose trust in them, follow them, and check on them.

You must know that you have lost mutual trust and respect by acting in this way.

Given that the body develops up until the age of twenty-one, it is necessary to know that a child's brain is alternately developing every two years until the age of twelve. Be patient with your children.

In the past thirty years, children with an incredibly large amount of positive energy have been born. They are called indigo children; such children did not know violence in their earlier incarnations, so they are extremely sensitive to negative energy in their environment. Be careful with children, love them and protect them.

Influence and Shaping of a Person between twelve and twenty-five Years of Age

People between the ages of twelve and twenty-five begin to think clearly. Therefore, parents or guardians cannot impose their will onto them anymore but need to adapt to a new situation. If you are a careful and gentle parent/guardian until your child is twelve years old, you will be able to talk to your child about all of their new life experiences, which is necessary for their further development and their understanding of the things surrounding them.

If you were not this kind of parent, you can expect smugness, arrogance, and aggression from your child. Do not be surprised if they retaliate; your child is simply giving back what it needed but did not get from you.

At this stage, the body matures. If you were a good parent or guardian, your child will appreciate it and ask you for advice.

If you were not, the child requires understanding and support from those around them. Children who are violent usually received negative energy from their parents, their rage and frustration from work, from unemployment, daily humiliations, and other things, and they become violent towards their friends and children from their class.

At this stage, the first groups of like-minded people, the first cliques and the first gangs appear. Children begin swearing, smoking, drinking alcohol, using drugs, having sex, engage in violence and fights and listen to loud music, but they do not understand that is not good for them, nor can they, given their limited knowledge of life.

Since everything that is harmful to the psychic or physical body carries negative energy, through consumption children lower the already small amount of energy they possess and destroy their young physical body, which has not yet fully developed. Consumption brings large-scale cell mutations and the development of diseases that can manifest on a physical level very quickly after consumption. Here we are not referring to vomiting after consuming alcohol or the hallucinations caused by drugs but to alcoholism and drug overuse that quickly develop because the young body is susceptible to changes.

The problem is first with the parents or guardians and then with the environment. Parents or guardians must want to help their child regardless of the fact that they mostly feel helpless and ashamed of their situation. Such refusal to understand a problem increases the already high level of negative energy and does not solve these problems. Such an attitude harms you and your child.

In terms of sexual activity that begins too early in life: nowadays a person's first sexual experience most frequently occurs under the influence of alcohol or drugs and is not connected to positive emotions. In addition, a common belief is that through this act a person enters the adult world and thereby becomes more mature. This is one of the wrong beliefs of today's world.

The problems that appear are diseases, although not necessarily sexually transmitted diseases. But the body reacts to the aggression caused by such irresponsible and selfish behavior. Such behavior signals to your body that you do not respect it, its development, or its slow maturing. Not without reason do people say that there is a time for everything. Positive emotions are necessary in everything, as they are in this case, and you need to know why you did something and for what reason, which concerns only you. Never do anything in your life because of other people that is not positive and directed primarily towards you and then towards others.

Since you did not resolve the majority of those primal urges with yourself, your body will constantly remind you of it, which means that you will frequently visit doctors. They will be happy to tell you that you can solve these problems by taking pills or something similar. You do not solve anything in doing so; you simply postpone things for later or resolve them in one of your future lives. Energy remains always, constantly, and forever.

Until you resolve the cause of negative energy in your physical body, it will follow you.

Swearing and derogatory words are nowadays one of the most widely spread problems. One swears because it is considered normal. It is not natural nor ever will be. Are you thinking about what you are saying to whom and what kind of ugly words you are pronouncing? The most common derogatory terms are for the male and female reproductive organs. One curses mostly about mothers who gave them life and without whom you would not have entered into a physical body and would not have learnt what you needed to learn. No matter how she behaved towards you, she is still your mother and you need to respect her. Derogatory words are used as buzzwords and because one is not skilled at expressing oneself, which means that one has a very scanty vocabulary. The problems occurring in today's society are mostly related to sexuality, relationships, intercourse, potency, and everything revolves around what you constantly mention in a derogatory sense. Energy you direct towards undermining and insulting sexuality is reflected in your sexual relations and partnerships. When you change that energy, your relationships will balance out as well.

Swear words used as buzzwords to curse the person that you are communicating with or to curse something or someone else – even when such communication is normal for your interlocutor and used frequently in speech in every sentence – denote a limited person. By communicating in such a way, people constantly insult themselves, vilify those around them, and show how little appreciation they have for themselves as well as others. This kind of behavior lowers your energy and is only accepted in groups of people who behave the same way. A group of such people is for the most part arrogant, smug, and aggressive.

One should remember the Lord's Ten Commandments.

1. I am the Lord your God. You shall not have other gods beside me (owing to God's consciousness, you are here on this Earth right now, in this time and this place).
2. You shall not invoke the name of the Lord in vain (when you speak about God, always speak with love).
3. Remember the Sabbath day – keep it holy (find time to spend in silence with your higher self).
4. Honor your father and your mother, that you may have a long life in the land the Lord your God is giving you (meaning God, because He is your father and mother).
5. You shall not kill.
6. You shall not commit adultery (swearing and unnatural intercourse; do not perform actions that lower your energy,
   since you are children of light).
7. You shall not steal.
8. You shall not bear false witness against your neighbor.
9. You shall not covet your neighbor's wife.

10. You shall not covet anything that belongs to your neighbor (because it lowers your energy and leads you away from your higher self).

Parents and guardians need to show children exactly how to behave and live by example. It is impossible to believe parents or guardians who tell their children that smoking or alcohol harms them while doing it themselves because it is senseless and selfish to do so before them. In such a way they are showing their children that they are immature, since it is known how harmful such consummation is for the physical body, and whilst doing it persistently, they are not respecting their children or their children's young bodies that are still developing (if they do it in front of them).They also show that they disregard life.

The differences among people fall into three groups. These are the roles: leader/follower, I do not want to be like them, and I do not fit into any group.

The first role, which is of the follower, means needing somebody to lead you because it makes you feel safe and protected. You lack energy, confidence and you are insecure. A leader is a person who has a lot of egoistic energy that feeds on the energy of his followers, and in such a way, he raises himself above the others, is smug, arrogant, and often aggressive, especially when a follower does not obey. Such situations are common in young people wanting to protect themselves from the insecurity they feel in their surroundings, whether in their family, school, or somewhere else. Adults get into such situations mostly when it comes to having their own way. (What is right is known only by God, because He knows all situations, all of your thoughts and the feelings that led you to it).

The second groups are people who do not want conflict, who do not want to argue or get their own way. They have more positive energy than the first group. They are particularly well-accepted in society because they can adapt to various situations.

The third group consists of younger people and is completely misunderstood and poorly accepted in society. If the family in which a child grows up does not have positive energy on a very high level, the child will feel completely misunderstood. Such people are scarce in the world, they are immensely positive, understand everybody, know how to give good advice, do not impose themselves, and will always help you selflessly and in the way that you need. Such people have an incredibly high level of positive energy; they are healthy emotionally and mentally. Later in life, people who still have not reached the point of wanting to improve their life find these positive people very repulsive and treat them rudely and want to hurt them, which is certainly impossible. Other people who have started down their paths towards truth are drawn to them like a magnet. Most people like this want to appropriate the positive person in some way, which is impossible. They are always at a natural distance because they do not get attached to people (attachment is a sign that you are still very connected to your physical body). Such people are free from all attachment and live in truth.

Think through everything you plan to do and whether it is good and positive for you. We all want to belong to a group until we realize that each individual always belongs to everybody and everything and that nobody has ever been separated from anything or anyone, because God made it so.

Parents and guardians, your children often want to belong to some group for protection. If they think that you cannot protect them, they find a way. Human beings are always in search of something good, something that can calm them and provide them with safety. Give your child what it needs. Talk about everything, not as a friend but as a parent. Do not act omniscient. You can learn a lot from your children and get rid of the frustrations imposed upon you by your parents or guardians. Listen to them, think sensibly, without yelling, rage, and misunderstanding and reach a solution together.

Influence and Shaping of a Person from the Age of twenty-five

From the age of twenty-five onwards people have for the most part already understood what is happening around them; they accept situations and try to sensibly and rationally affect what is happening to them and their surroundings.

By the age of twenty-five, the majority of people have accepted most of their frustrations and defined their way of thinking. In the next ten years of their lives, the only concern is what they will do for themselves in the material and emotional sense. After that, they are closed off to new possibilities, new solutions, and they limit themselves and forget how to live.

Frustrations imposed on you do not label you, except in cases where you accept them as a fact about your own personality. This means that you have accepted other people's way of thinking and other people's behavior as your own. You are not these things. They are them. You are what you are; you are what you were given at birth. It will always be so. It is up to you if you want to change it, or if you are satisfied with such a negative mental state. It means that you do not want to think about who you really are, you do not want to seek the truth, and you like being in other people's skins.

By accepting yourself as you are, you now, with your already-defined negative attitude, continuing on with your role as a martyr and sufferer full of self-pity. You think that you need to show others that they cannot play with you. Such an approach brings with it other negative emotions, aggression, smugness, and an increase in the ego. The ego is one of the strongest enemies to truth about the self. Ego shows the people around you that your individual "self" is completely separated from your selfhood, your true Source. Such people are usually aggressive, arrogant, distrustful, eloquent, and do not trust anyone but themselves.

Your arrogance is pushing people away, you think that you are in a circle of the chosen ones and such a role suits you. The question is, until when? Most egoistic people are afraid to think about it, let alone search for a cause and solution.

Such a relationship towards yourself makes you a closed-off person, immune to what is happening around you. You think that by reopening, by accepting people again, someone might hurt you once more, and you run away from it.

Given this attitude towards the self, and since you entered into a physical body in order to develop and overcome the problems that you need to understand in this life, you happen to constantly repeat similar situations in life. This means that you have not solved your problem; instead, you repeat the same pattern of behavior all over again. Until you stop and think about why some things in your life are constantly repeating, you will get yourself into more and more difficult situations, and in the end, you will not have the power or the will to fight. Life is not a struggle but rather learning through various roles. You are an actor, and how you play the role is up to you.

Due to their numerous frustrations, people do not know how to communicate with one another. A simple conversation about the weather becomes a quarrel. You can say anything in a conversation, but first you have to think about the person you are communicating with in terms of their character and their ability to understand and comprehend. You have to understand that this way of communicating is good for you and that it makes you feel good. Afterwards, be aware of your words and the tone of your voice. In other words, everything can be said, but you have to be careful how, in order for the conversation to be a conversation and not turn into something unwanted. When you pay attention to it for some time, you will realize that it makes you feel better because understanding others makes you understand that you are accepting your differences as well. Similarly, it will become acceptable behavior, and after some time, you will not need to think, but you will have a presentiment and know how to communicate. Certainly, sometimes you just need to keep quiet and listen to your interlocutor; irrespective of the fact that it is a monologue, it is a form of communication too.

Many people claim that they will never change, that they are old enough, and that change is for younger people. They believe they are fulfilled, mature enough have enough life experience, and that such an attitude, knowledge, and behavior can help younger people to correctly realize themselves. If you do not possess inner peace and you cannot stay completely calm in each situation you face, you have more to learn. Making changes does not refer solely to young people but to everybody. Making changes does not mean altering attitudes but altering yourselves, understanding yourselves. Only when people understand themselves can they completely understand the situation around them, carefully review it, tell themselves that they have understood, and move on. Understanding your environment and the circumstances around you, and understanding other people and their actions, changes you. You are altered in a positive direction and slowly come to understand the truth about yourself. You are now, at this moment, in an altered state; it is necessary to comprehend that and bring yourself into the right state that makes you feel safe, calm, full of understanding, peace, and love towards the self and others. Then you can help anyone who asks you to because you are energetically bound to a higher knowledge, your consciousness.

Alcoholism is a very common affliction these days because people fall into mourning for their very selves. Such people love when others feel sorry for them and they enjoy such a role. Your alcoholism is nobody's fault. Alcoholics always look for a reason to drink. Doctors say that alcoholism is present in every second generation of a family. You look for an excuse everywhere apart from within. What is inherited and accepted is an energetic behavioral pattern that can go from generation to generation, but not alcoholism as such. If your grandfather was an alcoholic because he felt sorry for himself, because he knew he would be left alone and he could do whatever crossed his mind, the alcoholic inherited the energy of feeling sorry for themselves and other patterns but not the alcoholism (the addiction itself). Does it suit you that alcohol constantly destroys your brain cells and that you become forgetful or aggressive towards your loved ones, who experience frustration because of you, just because you can support your feeling of pity towards self? You think that it is fine on your side.

Nowadays it is commonplace for the doctor to find a cure for all your problems. You see a doctor, he examines you in the best way he can, which means your physical body. In any case, your frustrations are absolutely diagnostically irrelevant to him, as are your feelings of self-pity, insecurity, feelings of inadequacy, hate, and others. He, of course, knows what is wrong with you, and you are overjoyed because you will get some pill that will rid you of the problems you nurtured and embraced for years, just like that. When it is suppressed, suddenly after some time, the same problem recurs but with more intensity, perhaps not in the exact same spot, but in another. What then? Do you go to the same or to another doctor and so on and so forth until you need surgery? What then? They persuade you nicely that it is the only way to survive and they dissociate themselves by making you sign some agreement prior to the surgery and tell you that they do not know whether the disease will return or not.

At the beginning of the 1960s, people began living more intensely, faster, and more unhealthily than before. Then a great and fast exchange of energies had begun, not only in people but in their relationships as well. Doctors who observed human beings from the physical body's point of view (which is mostly how it is done today as well) needed to adapt to a new situation, which is not the case now because then there would be more psychiatrists and psychologists. Nowadays it is still embarrassing to see a psychiatrist or a psychologist, but it is not shameful to jeopardize and bully your closest ones because of your frustrations. Make a move; it is up to you. Do something positive for yourself in order to help yourself and those around you.

No one can tell you whether you correctly defined the problem that caused the diseased state you are in because you are perfectly aware of it. You just need to be open towards yourself and you will realize this. A wish to be open towards yourself will motivate you to try and find a solution for your problem. The best and the only solution is asking your higher consciousness, which is located in your heart, for an answer. The most appropriate time is right before falling asleep because then your consciousness is the most open to questions directed towards your heart, and your physical body is relaxed. If you are indeed willing to find out the truth, it will be given to you. That is why it is said, ask and you shall receive.

Changing partners frequently is very common these days. Perhaps it is normal for society today, but it is not natural. People who are unstable and do not know what they want from themselves and others constantly change partners and continuously hope they will find the missing piece of themselves. Of course, it will not happen in this way. It is also common, in order to forget your old relationship, that you head into a new one in order to reduce your pain, sorrow, insecurity, and loss. You do not fix anything in doing so; the same things happen to you, only with another person. It means that you have not considered why you constantly seek out people with similar or the same personality traits. These are mostly people who can display the traits of one of your parents very convincingly. Does that suit you? Do not rush. Take your time. By not taking your time to think, you lower your energy and the energy of the person you are with because you cannot give that person understanding and acceptance if you have not found those feelings within yourself, let alone lived them. Better to be alone with yourself for some time than to do harm to another.

Partners are usually sexual partners. Some people see themselves as irresistible, narcissistic, and want to prove to themselves that they are still wanted, which in fact has nothing to do with their view of themselves but rather with a desire to get support from those around them. Firstly, you never need to prove anything to anyone, let alone yourself, especially not in that way. Sexual energy is one of the strongest energies apart from the energy of love and fear; after all, it enables the creation of new life. Playing with it, which is mostly done by those who have affairs and those who often change partners, is very dangerous. Every person you have physical contact with, you will eventually have to meet and resolve your relationship. It is very likely that you will have to work out that part in one of your future lives. Therefore, think about what you are doing, everything has its cause and effect.

Adultery is also common nowadays. Since I mentioned that sexual energy is one of the strongest energies, all sexual partners carry a small part of that energy from another person. Besides, most people are intuitive, which means that they sense changes in the energy field of their partners and unconsciously know when their partner is cheating on them. No one can be cheated on except for you yourself. By cheating, you show your immaturity, insecurity, egoism, detachment from yourself, and your wish to stand out, which in any case decreases your energy and leads to diseases.

If you want to end a relationship and your partner does not want to, when it comes to the roles of tyrant/victim or the desire to possess, there is a solution for everything. Be patient; ask God for help. The higher consciousness will always respond to your requests; no matter how hard it is, send love and forgiveness to these kinds of people. By increasing your energy there is an automatic release from the current situation, so your partner will want to end the relationship by themselves. Be patient and send love to yourself and the other person.

In violent situations, do not hesitate to ask for help right away, and be led by love – because only then will everything be resolved in the way that is best for you and the other person – so that you will be protected.

It is important to realize that you are responsible for everything that happens after the age of twenty-five. Up until then, your parents, guardians, and your environment were responsible. Assume responsibility for yourself and do not place the blame on others. Blaming others means not accepting the truth that you create your own destiny. That is why it is said that every man is the master of his own destiny. It is said that your destiny is guaranteed at birth. It is not destiny but what you must learn during your life. You build your own path and destiny with your thoughts, in other words, with your attitudes and goals.

How you behave and speak of others reflects what you actually think about yourself.

It is interesting how everyone would like to solve their problems quickly, even though they planted them, nurtured them, and took care of them for years. If you want to solve them, be patient, be determined, and have faith. You have to know and want to find a cause in order to solve a consequence, a disease.

Maturity means accepting truth and living in truth, behaving correctly, accepting what we are, living in peace, understanding ourselves and our environment, and living in love, out of love, and for love.

When you rise above, to a greater extent your energy is purified and you become immune to external negative influences because you realize that people you meet on a daily basis have yet to learn a lot, to walk the same path but in their own way like you did, and you consider them young people regardless of their age.

Commitment is an act of love. It is a belief that the power of love can achieve anything, even when you cannot foresee the final outcome of a situation, which is usually the case. With commitment, ego is lost, there is only “I am”. It is a quest for your higher self and faith in truth. In order to give yourself to love and live in truth, you need to reject the ego, your physical “I”.

You should do and say only what is in your interest and the interests of those around you. If anything is harmful in any way, whether for you or those around you, near or far, it is not right, and you should give it up right away. Perhaps at this moment it is not appropriate, but it will be when the situation is right. Sometimes this never happens, and you realize that things turned out for the best for everyone involved.

You should be able to tell your parents everything in an acceptable way, and it is up to them to accept it and realize why you said things in such a way and what the purpose of your tone is. They should learn something through such conversation.

When a person talks to another person or multiple people, one can realize according to the volume and color of their voice what kind of person they are and how much they care for the other people they are communicating with. When your voice is quiet, you are in an excellent relationship with that person; you understand each other well and are supportive, even though you are not aware of it in your verbal communication. Your hearts are close. When you have a loud conversation with people, you strive to reach those people because you realize that, otherwise, they would not receive your verbal message. Your hearts are very distant from one another.

How to Free Yourself from Frustration

Everything exists and happens for a reason. There is not anything that happens that does not have its purpose or function. Therefore, you must observe, perceive, and accept everything as it is. Observe everything like you are an actor or an actress on stage, unbiased. It will help you understand the purpose and function of everything happening around you.

UNDERSTAND whether you want to change your life or not. Does such a way of life suit you? Did you accept it so much that you consider it truly yours?

If you realize that you cannot go on like this, you have to decide whether you are willing to change everything in order to feel better and live differently than you do now.

Then you make the DECISION that you truly want to change something in your life, but do not understand what. Most people know how they would like to live, but do not dare to take the first step, because afterwards, of course, there are other steps. After you decide, the whole Universe, positive energy, will be directed towards helping you in your endeavor to realize your goals if they are good for you, or to solve your life's mission or some part of it. Since everyone has their wishes, hopes and expectations, it is necessary to FOCUS on a desired change. Start listening to what you say and start noticing what you do and why you do it, what affected the things you do in a certain way and DEFINE YOUR GOAL.

Define your goal by writing your wishes down on a piece of paper. Each wish, or goal, should be written in a positive sense as if it is happening right now, in the present. For instance, "I have a person that I love and who loves me by my side, I have beautiful and clever children, I live happily, I have everything I need, I have peace and joy, I am healthy..."

Considering the fact that when you start thinking in this way and solving situations in your life, you actually do not have any real guidelines and strength, the simplest way is to ask someone you trust for help. They will certainly help you. The best and the most acceptable way is to refer to a saint or some holy person from your religion. Be adamant; repeat your wishes every day. When you convince yourself that you truly want it, help will come instantaneously because at that moment you have created a connection between yourself and your higher "I". You can pray anywhere or go to church when it is empty.

It is of utmost importance to know what the PURPOSE of your life is. Some people have a complex, and others a simpler, purpose in life. Every purpose has a positive direction. One's purpose can be, for instance, wanting to be a good and self-sacrificing parent or guardian or wanting to be your nation's leader for the greater good. It can happen that the purpose you were given is lived out in a negative sense, which occurs because in coming to the Earth people receive free will, and most come having completely forgotten what their purpose on Earth is.

Pay attention to what you think, want, and hope for because all energy remains permanently marked.

What you do in this life, the way you live, the way you treat others and yourself; it all leaves a trace on this life of yours. Nothing is lost, and that is why frustration and stress occur. Therefore, it is necessary to ANALYZE YOURSELF as a person, everything you have been carefully collecting during your life.

It is necessary to define and understand frustration and stress, define the feelings related to frustration and stress, and define your current health problems on a physical level because they are connected to the frustrations and stresses you have been through. In order to do that, you need to define:

- how your parents or guardians treated you during your childhood

We are here referring to their actions, attitudes, conversations, and their violent behavior towards the gentle psyche of children, which can be described as saying things, such as:

- how could you not know that, everybody knows that
- how can you be so irresponsible
- you never use your head; I won't always think instead of you
- let them – you are older
- let them – you are smarter
- how could this happen to you

- you are really careless
- your insolent behavior has crossed the line
- I haven't taught you that
- if you don't tell me you'll be sorry
- from whom did you inherit that – not from me
- you must not do that; it is not good for you
- you don't understand that

When parents or guardians underestimate a child or impose a sense of guilt, it results in a child becoming cynical, feeling worthless, feeling hurt, becoming small-minded, defiant, rebellious, bitter, limited, big-headed, or egoistic. In addition, parents and guardians can be physically violent along with those insults, so a child becomes estranged and isolated, has a wish to disappear or to cease to exist, is deeply hurt, feels unworthy of love, attention and understanding, and feels hate and anxiety.

There is also another relevant way to behave and speak that can send a person in an unwanted direction, and parents or guardians think that they are directed in the most positive sense for their child:

- my child is the best
- you are the smartest
- this person is not worthy of you
- we are all listening to you
- you give the best advice
- we will give you everything
- you are our most beloved child

Most such parents or guardians give children money or support without real positive feelings. Then it happens that people become egocentric and arrogant, underestimate others, or become enraged and aggressive, and other aforementioned traits.

Your parents' or guardians' actions should not be justified but understood.

- the way your parents or guardians treated each other while you were living with them

You are also defined by the way your parents treated each other, since all energy surrounding them was always reaching you because you were mostly near them. Simply by observing, all their quarrels, insults, their showing of positive emotions, whether they treated each other with respect or not, physical violence from a parent or a guardian, underestimating a parent or guardian, you define your view of these things. Later you imposed these things on your relationships with the people around you, your partners, and the people you work with.

- the way they treat you now (when you are older and not as emotionally attached to them)

If they still act like people who continually want you to adapt to their way of thinking and their behavior, treating you as a person who can still be shaped according to their wishes and frustrations.

- the way their parents treated them

Since all parents or guardians have their own frustrations, they actually live out the frustrations of their parents or guardians. It used to be deeply rooted and now it is the case that mothers know everything and must be listened to without question. There used to be fewer deep emotions than now. Your parents or guardians mostly live out the behavior of their parents; one must be the head of the house and finances are handled by only one person, while another does not know even what is going on; one is a handyman around the house, and there is a division of male and female work.

When you have reassessed everything, write it down. Take a piece of paper and write down your frustration on the left side of the paper. Put the emotions they caused and how they affect you as a person in the middle. On the right side you need to write down positive statements. At the end of the list write what kind of health-related problems you have. It should, for instance, look like this:

shame	a parent or a guardian says you should be ashamed of yourself, what you are doing, why are you eating like that, what are you wearingfeelings of insecurity and running away from people	I support myself and everything that I do is in harmony with myself

health: stomach issues

isolation	a parent or a guardian avoided me because their work was more important than meI felt less worthy and began to avoid running into them	I am happy among people and they accept me

health: a lump in the throat, facial redness, stiffness

You have reassessed what you could recall, which was deeply repressed for many years. Most of these things you did not even wish to recollect because you thought that you cannot change anything anyway. What is done is done, but it is necessary to recall it in order to cleanse yourself of the accumulated negative energy and become free.

After defining and understanding the situation comes ACCEPTING ONESELF with all one's frustrations and stresses because they are an indelible part of life. After acceptation of yourself as you are now comes UNDERSTANDING ONESELF, since you could not affect what happened to you in your youth or change it. One of the biggest problems is that you need to try and understand your parents and guardians because they did not know how to change their situation and how to understand it later in order to avoid mistakes while they were raising you. When you realize what happened in your life and with your life, you should be able to FORGIVE. To forgive means to realize the truth about your life that has shaped you, realize that what happened cannot be changed. Nor is it necessary because in that way, you were given a chance to learn and rise above each situation that will occur in the future. You will, considering your understanding of your earlier life, be able to define it and solve it. In doing so you realize how connected to yourself and your omniscient higher "self" you are.

Until you realize why, some situations and events repeatedly occur in your life, with time often even more intensely. They will repeat because you have created a pattern in your life that you do not want to get rid of, and it is connected to the purpose you need to fulfill in this life towards yourself.

All situations in the future will be understood and resolved quickly. You will realize that everything that happened to you before has determined who you are as a person, which means that now you can define yourself, your personality, and the life you want in the future. You will realize that most situations do not necessarily need to happen to you in order for you to understand life and to develop as a person, but it is enough simply to observe situations, the people in them, their emotions and reactions.

When it comes to your energy and your desires, events are created from which you need to learn something. You will realize that, when you understand yourself, you will relax and tell yourself that it is not necessary to repeat the situation in its previous – or any other – form because you understand the situation that happened or was happening to you.

Since you understand yourself and your parents or guardians, you can understand all other people on Earth. Everybody needs to deal with similar events, similar situations, and needs to learn the same way you did because it is everybody's goal to understand and grow in Love. Nobody should be pitied, but simply state the situation and understand it. Everything that happens, happens for a reason, and the goal is one and the same for everyone. Only the paths are different. The path you choose depends on what you mean to resolve with your reincarnation in this life, what your purpose is. After that, you are shaped by your parents or guardians, until you are twenty-five. Later everything is up to you.

Since parents' or guardians' behavior and speech cause negative energy in a child, when the time comes that a child wants to change it because it cannot live like that anymore, firstly it needs to get rid of that negative energy in order to focus on receiving, and accepting life with positive energy. It is a long and painful process, but it is inevitable.

You are not determined by words or the behavior of your parents or guardians. If you were told that you will not achieve anything if you do not finish university, or you will never have money because they are poor, it has nothing to do with you. You are a unique individual and so you should behave, but always in harmony with love, and you will never do wrong. By refusing to accept their way of life, you clear your energy field of their negative energies.

Given that accumulated negative energy in a child's energy field causes various frustrations, as well as unnatural, inappropriate, and unacceptable behavior, it also causes situations and events in their environment when an adult considers things difficult and feels as if somebody is punishing them. Such situations are mostly similar to situations that the person lived through as a child. Now, as an adult, it is necessary to confront them, realize them, and understand them in order for them to stop repeating. By understanding situations from one's childhood that a child at a young age cannot influence, a person changes and raises their energy field to a higher level. Until people appreciate why such situations happen, they will constantly enter the same situations that were given to them in order to understand that part of their lives and what should have happened, regardless of how difficult it was.

In such situations it is usually said that a son chooses a wife based on her character, sometimes even based on her looks, which are similar to those of his mother, or that a daughter finds a man who is in many respects similar to her father.

Forgetting is something that parents or guardians often mention; forget how I acted towards you, you are an adult now, forget that you were beaten, mistreated, insulted. Nobody can forget anything, ever, because all that is energy remains permanently marked. There is no forgetting, only understanding and forgiveness in order to reach the truth.

When you reach a degree of understanding yourself and the situations and events around you, you usually want to help others realize what you achieved within yourself. First you reach out to those who are closest to you, which is usually your close and extended family. If there is a misunderstanding, the conclusion is that they do not care to be better off, they are not yet ready for change, and that it is not yet time to accept the fact that there is something better beyond their limited world. Such people should then be left alone with their explanations because they lead nowhere. The only thing you can give those people, as well as everyone else around you, is understanding and love.

Do not judge and argue because you do not know what made the person you are observing act that way. It is said; judge not lest ye be judged. Since people are very keen on judging others simply to avoid thinking about themselves, their behavior, and actions, they turn to another person who is usually energetically weaker and is judged based on their own experiences. Since people have their own different experiences and accept them and understand them in their own way, it is very likely that all judgments are absolutely subjective and do not have anything to do with truth.

Being polite and calm, regardless of the situation, is very important. In this way you show people around you that you understand them and are striving to accept them however they may present themselves. Until people realize that they are not what other people or the media that shaped them for years made of them, but that they are children of God, you can only observe, try to help, and always and in every moment be polite, regardless of how difficult it may sometimes be.

It is imperative to thank everyone and for everything. Thanks needs to come from your heart and not just be pronounced without feeling. With the help of thanking from your heart, you raise your energy, and you, as well as the person you are thankful to, are fulfilled.

The things that you say of others and to others, and whether you behave according to your words, are the opinions you hold of yourself. In other words, if you underestimate someone or are angry towards them, you actually underestimate yourself and do not consider yourself a person worthy of attention and respect. You do not like it at all, so such dissatisfaction is transferred on other people who have less energy than you.

It is sometimes a problem to give advice because you do not know details about a person's life, you do not know what they need to learn in this life and do not know if that person is ready to listen to your advice. Besides, how certain are you that you are competent enough to talk about certain issues and to solve those issues in the right way? If you want to give advice to someone and you know that the person expects it and will listen to you, first connect to your higher "self", which means that you need to be completely calm and listen to that person without bias and with lots of love and understanding in your heart. Most people listen with their emotions, feelings, and the experiences they have in life. It is then that you usually give bad advice and make the wrong decisions in life. When you are connected to your all-knowing and ever-present higher "self", you always make the right decisions for your own good and the good of those around you.

It is now clear that God does not punish anyone. It is up to you; you define everything with your thoughts. If you want to be happy, you already are, and you just need to realize it. If you want to be sad, you already are since you defined yourself as such.

God is not here to be addressed with awe. You are here thanks to Him and He leads you through your life like a real parent. When He sees that you have wandered from your path (and everyone has their own), He will warn you. You are not sinners but children of God who strive for unity with their parent, that is, to return to your God.

When you connect to your higher "self," your life becomes easier because you have accepted what you were often told: worries and problems should be given to God. In doing so, you find a way out of all life's situations in a simple and painless way. At any given moment you know what you should do and how. What is best for you and for the good of the people around you is that you stop living in fear and start living the truth.

Let yourself go and go with the flow but keep your eyes wide open because life is beautiful.

Respect everyone and thank God and other people for everything.

There are situations that occur in your life that cannot be explained or connected to events or situations from this life. Often, they are phobias. This is energy that we brought with us into this life in order to resolve it, and it is related to one or more situations we lived through but did not understand or accept in one or more of our previous lives. If such energy is given to you in this life, it means that you can resolve it because everything that enters this life and is brought with you is brought because you knew that you could resolve it in this life. It is also one of the purposes for which you came to this world.

Changes that occur by changes to your thoughts and through an understanding of previous situations and forgiveness cannot be expressed in words. An attitude such as this changes your energy. It becomes pure, lighter, and stronger, and your whole body is healthier, until you are completely healthy. Being healthy and living healthily does not only mean eating healthy but living healthily in Love with yourself and those around you.

It can be felt intensely in your environment. Those people who followed your path, those who want to but do not know how, or those who need positive energy will soon appear near you, which will for the most part confuse you.

People from your family will be confused by your new energy, as well as your attitude towards yourself or them. Most do not tolerate such changes because they are confused and, they do not realize the change that occurred and how to behave in a new situation. You will be met with rejection, angry outbursts, and under-estimation, but they will, at the same time, ask to be near you because you will make them feel comfortable and calm. Such behavior will surely last for some time, maybe even longer, depending on their energy level. If they will not adapt to a new situation, there will be disagreement in thought, quarrels will occur, and you will not share a common language anymore. You will need to part ways, which will be painful for both sides, but you will feel relieved. Given that they are your family, they will eventually accept these changes, and your relationship will be more harmonious than ever. By accepting your changes, they have accepted the possibility of changing themselves so that their energy will grow and harmonize with yours. They will then become more satisfied, happier, and healthier.

When people around you accept your positive changes, they will see that you have become happier, calmer and healthier, that you accept your environment easily, and that you deal with new events and situations with ease, and they will be more joyful and happier with you. You not only help yourself by increasing your positive energy, but that of the people around you too, and your relationship becomes more harmonious and much healthier.

When it comes to friendships, you usually socialize with people who are on more or less the same frequency as you, which means that your energies are compatible and support each other. Since you will grow in positive energy, there will be great positive changes in your energy field, which will confuse your former friends. Those who will not be able to adapt to your new positive energy will simply grow distant from you because you will not have any common interests. The part of life you shared with them and grew through with them has ended, and you will part ways. Do not grieve. They were here for you and because of you, as you were there for them and because of them. Think about what you needed to go through with those people, what your mutual support was like, and what you learned from that relationship. After that, new people will enter your life, and they will be compatible with your new energy, so you will get along well with them in an excellent way and exchange your life experiences in a more positive manner.

This refers to romantic relationships as well. There are people who constantly search for themselves. As soon as they begin traveling down their own path with a goal, they find direction. If a person cannot follow their partner's path, they will split up.

Do not lay claim to anyone; every single person is an individual; nobody is anyone's property, nor will they ever be. An attitude such as this shows the people around you how insecure you are, how alone you feel, and how you need someone to fill the emptiness in your life, which means that you are distant from your selfhood, from your true "self". If you cannot accept and endure yourself, why do you think that someone else has to? Confront yourself and realize that the things you constantly search for in others are actually within you but that you have repressed them deeply. Let them out onto the surface and let them envelop you, and then you will feel free to enter into healthy relationships and partnerships, not only with friends and family but with your romantic partner as well.

Everyone has their moment. When that moment comes, there is a decision to be made and a quest for truth, for the revelation of your true selfhood. Do not force anyone to understand because they will not; that particular person has yet to reach this moment. Have patience for everyone around you because they all eventually take that path, since it is a goal that everybody is searching for.

After increasing your positive energy, other things will catch your interest, you will be captivated by things that never crossed your mind. You will start noticing people, things, events, accepting them as they are because it is necessary in order to understand them and because they were caused by people due to their way of thinking, their attitudes, and behavior.

The positive energy you will attract will affect the changing of your wishes with respect to other people. You will want to do good deeds, to help from the bottom of your heart, to be attentive, gentle, and understanding, and it will fill your heart endlessly. You will feel fulfilled, like you are finally living, because one of your tasks is to fulfill yourself by giving love through good deeds.

By increasing and strengthening your positive energy you will again conjure your intuition to lead you and direct you. It is only necessary for you to recognize it. And so, you will, because everything happening with you and around you give you the feeling that it is positive when it comes to you and your environment. After that, let it guide you. Listen carefully to your body; it knows everything in order for you to catch the signs it is sending you in time. Signs are always like a warning. Most commonly they relate to people you meet and need to communicate with, and very often they concern some events, regardless of whether they are of a personal or a business nature. Your body can warn you perfectly well whether to work with a certain person or not, to take that path or to stay home. Listen to it.

Everything will then be directed towards the realization of your newest needs, but on a higher, more positive energy level. Such an attitude towards the self will cause more positive people to enter your life, positive life changes (such as a new partner if you find it necessary), new friends, new employment, a new, more positive work environment. If you are unemployed, you will get a job; if you do not have a partner, and you want one, you will get one (but pay attention to how you characterize them, because that is what you will get), or you will get health or money.

It is said that money changes people. Because of that attitude, people do not have money. If you are negatively directed towards a need, in this case money, then you are constantly pushing it away. It is like that with everything. If you are convinced that people can get a job only through connections, then you will not get it, or you will get it that way. If you are convinced that your partner will behave like one of your parents or guardians, then you will receive such a partner. If you are convinced that you are perfect (and you are not, because if you were, you would not think of yourself in such a way) and that you are always right (your attitude shows that you are not), you will always get into situations that will show you that you are wrong and lead you to conflicts.

Pay attention to what you imagine and how positive your thoughts are, because it will happen. Everything is energy as long as you move it using your thoughts, and if you are really focused on it, it will happen.

You will realize what living a lie means. A lie is not only a false truth as people see it, the twisting and imagining of events and situations that happen to people. A lie is also not understanding the truth as a human being, the truth you receive when you are born, the truth about what being human means: how one should live, why and how to behave, and how to be what you are. By understanding the truth about what a person is, one stops living a lie.

People usually lie to protect themselves. Since that is the way to justify yourself and the lies that bring others pain, insecurity, or other negative feelings, such attitudes harm people because as it has been said, what goes around comes around. Very often events and reverse situations happen, and a person then loses trust in themselves and other people. It does not bring anyone any good.

If you want to get out of a situation, always tell the truth; whether it is only half of it or the whole is up to you. With half-truths that are still truths, you always let the other person choose what to conclude about your truth.

When you define and determine everything, let go, but from time to time pay attention to the course of your life so you can redirect it towards the correct path – the one you took – and take your time. There is always enough time, regardless of how old you are, because age is defined solely by your physical body, not your spiritual one. The soul is eternal; it has always been, it is so now, and so it shall always be.

As soon as you start finding truth and living in truth, it will get easier when you reenter the karmic pattern and reincarnate somewhere else in some other place and some other time.

Given that everyone is an individual carrying their own energy, there is nothing beyond that energy.

Given that everything around us is energy, visible or invisible, there is nothing beyond that energy.

Given that we and everything that was created are connected with energy, there is nothing beyond that energy.

Given that everything, animate and inanimate, visible and invisible, was created from that energy, there is nothing beyond that energy.

Given that everything is energy, we are all inter-connected and communicate amongst ourselves through energy, there is nothing beyond that energy.

PART III

How Thoughts, Behavior and Feelings Work

Inner dissatisfaction with the world we live in and judging other people causes migraines, head trauma, meningitis, and diseases of the nasal mucosa. If you do not change the way you think, there is an assault on the genitor-urinary system.

When a person judges a lot and has bad thoughts, the liver suffers. If a person insults others or is angry and has strong reactions, there can be damage to the heart.

The stomach is damaged when a person is often angry and insults not only those that are closest to them but themselves as well (cursing). The reason is dissatisfaction with the outside world and their destiny, as well as constant inner rejection to accepting situations in life.

Fear can block the physical body. There are events in life after which you constantly experience the same or similar situations. In order to overcome and surpass this, recall the situation and try to resolve it. For example, children get into a fight, a children's fight without physical consequences, but the boy who should have won the fight suddenly froze with fear and lost. It is considered a serious pathological disorder, but such a situation would disappear if the boy were alone, which means that if he was in a risky situation where he is the only participant, fear would not occur. Fear appears only when he needs to show resistance to someone. He was further abused after that situation, and he showed no resistance. It is a feeling of being unprotected, which is gained in youth from one's parents or guardians.

Fear can lead to sudden death, so in each situation, no matter how difficult and hopeless it seems, you should be calm because you are connected to an omniscient energy in doing so. Remain open and listen to your inner voice.

Only true love is an inexhaustible source of energy. If people are hopeless and critical in some situations, they forget about ephemeral values in life and turn to limitless love, so they will always find the right solution. Then people can do wonders. Physical healing is a small part of that.

People who reject love lead themselves into deadly situations, such as incurable diseases (which at their core do not exist), accidents with difficult repercussions and other forms of self-destruction, or even death.

If you were in love, after a separation or a break-up there should be joy in your heart because of the fact that you met each other at all and for the joyful moments you shared and not the bitterness of the end.

Lung cancer can occur in people who got used to relying upon themselves, their abilities, and their reasoning ever since they were children. Such people usually succeed in what they had planned to do. As long as they rely on their abilities, they find themselves in situations in which they have difficulty accepting the inconveniences and mishaps around them. After some time, they put a lot of effort into controlling situations in life, and by that, they forget that they should learn something from all situations and that these are given to them to realize that they should not treat themselves that way.

Cancer is a disease caused by deep bitterness hiding within a person for a long time until it literally eats away at their body. Usually there is an event in childhood that destroys trust in life. Such an experience is never forgotten. Such people live with a feeling of self-pity. They are unable to develop and maintain meaningful and long-term romantic relationships. Such people see their lives as a series of disappointments. The feeling of hopelessness, helplessness, and loss overtake such people's thoughts and they blame others for all the problems in their lives. People who have cancer are self-critical. In order to cure cancer, it is necessary to accept and love yourself.

The cause of asthma is excessive conspicuity and a feeling of personal importance, as well as a craving for life, a desire for and awareness of life. Asthma occurs only in people who tell themselves that they do not have the right to breathe, the right to enjoy life. Consequently, one should not fight against nature but adapt.

Asthma occurs in children who have a strongly developed consciousness and they consider themselves responsible for the events that occur in their environment. They feel worthless and helpless, and they assume guilt and are prone to self-punishment. Attacks can decrease and disappear during their development and as they grow up, but there is a possibility that in adulthood some experiences will trigger an unresolved situation from one's childhood, so the person will experience another episode of asthma, which can worsen through the years. In that way, they unconsciously relive a situation or situations from their childhood.

Bronchitis usually coincides with anger and blame. Since it is good to get anger and rage out of yourself, it is better to do so by breaking an object than inflicting physical and mental consequences on someone. By getting rid of one's anger and rage there is a smaller chance of contracting diseases. Strive to understand when it happened in order to understand the situation that continues to recur. The cause needs to be resolved in order to cure the consequences (rage, anger).

People usually use reason and logic to judge things happening around them, thereby forgetting about the thoughts and feelings that created them. If feelings do not provide enough security for adapting to a new situation, conscious reasoning loses its ground becomes insecure, and there is uncertainty and fear. For example, people who have repeatedly been in traffic accidents where there is only material damage still feel insecurity while driving. Your emotional state while driving is connected to possible inconveniences constantly occurring to you in your mind. If you have bad thoughts about pedestrians, it is possible to run over a person; thoughts directed towards traffic officers, driving itself, or parked cars usually cause this. Similarly, ostentation and arrogance in driving are a direct way to get into an accident or commit suicide. Your emotional state determines what your driving will be like. When an accident does occur, it determines the scope of the accident; long before it happens, everything is first defined in your thoughts.

Jealous people often suffer from weak circulation in their hands and legs. If it is related to human relationships and reaches the level of dependence on others to whom you are very attached, reproach can damage your eyesight.

Diabetes is a disease that can appear when you begin killing the love within you because you were previously hurt by a person you loved deeply. Stress remains in your body after a separation or divorce until we accept that situation and forgive ourselves and others.

Hair loss occurs with tension and fear. Tension is mostly felt in the shoulders, and it raises towards the top of one's head, hence the problem with facial muscle contraction. It causes great tension in the scalp; it condenses so hair cannot breathe, and it dies and falls off. If the scalp is not relaxed, new hair cannot grow. If you have gotten rid of the tension, the problem with hair growth reduction could lie in clogged follicles (pores) as well. Feeling tension is a sign of weakness. If you cannot relax your entire body, at least you try to relax your scalp. Gentle massage is always welcome.

Headaches occur when people are punishing themselves. Ask yourself what the reason behind it is, forgive yourself, and you will be free of it. Migraines occur in people who are under self-inflicted pressure. It includes a lot of suppressed rage.

Sinus issues in people are usually caused by being irritated by a close person. The problem with such people is that they blame others for their frustrations. Not one person, place, or thing has power over us because we are the ones who affect our bodies through our thoughts.

The throat represents the ability to say what we think. People with throat problems feel unable to stand up for themselves. A sore throat always means that a person has repressed rage.

The breasts represent your attitude towards relationships. Breast problems usually occur due to excessive feelings towards a person, place, thing, or experience. Similarly, they can occur due to rejection of the maternal in a woman, abortion, the rejection of your own child, negligence, and alienation. With breast cancer there is a deep bitterness towards one's attitudes and principles.

The heart represents love, and blood represents joy. When people deny themselves love, there is decreased blood flow so pain in the heart area occurs, as well as a heart attack. People who have suffered a heart attack usually do not get joy out of life.

Bladder issues usually occur in people who are, as romantic partners, very bitter. They are usually angered by something connected to femininity or masculinity. Women have bladder problems more often than men because they are more prone to hiding that they have been hurt.

Issues with the vagina usually show that a woman feels emotionally hurt by her partner. Prostate issues are related to self-respect and the belief that the man is less and less competent as he ages.

Loss or absence of potency lies in a wish to subdue women, unconscious aggression, thoughts directed solely towards physical needs and pleasure, and being directed towards looking at and flirting with the female sex, as well as excessive sex fantasies. Impotence includes fear, sometimes disdain, towards the previous lover.

Frigidity happens out of fear and disdain towards the self, as well as due to an insensitive partner.

The colon represents the ability of the body to free itself from what it does not need anymore. Every body has its own rhythm. If the body is not in harmony with its rhythm, there are digestion issues. Similarly, people fear loss (piling up things they do not want to get rid of), and do things that smother them or do not afford themselves any pleasures because they need to put money away for a rainy day.

Obesity can occur due to the excessive consumption of food. Think a little: do you actually need to burden your body unnecessarily, including your internal organs and spine, by continuously adding mass to your body? The simplest way is to have your urine tested for acidity and alkalinity. Check the level of acidity. Everything beyond the optimum amount shows that you eat too much acidic food. In that case, eat foods that are alkaline and vice versa. In order to bring your body into balance and reach your optimal weight, eat foods that enable this, which means that it is necessary to make sure that the foods you eat are less acidic, but more alkaline.

Obesity represents a need for protection. People seek protection to avoid being hurt, belittled, criticized, cheated, or having a fear of living. Usually people who feel insecure and uncomfortable eat excessively in order to restore safety through eating. No diet will help you lose weight. The only way is to realize why you are insecure and why you are seeking comfort in food. When you put your body into balance, your weight will decrease by itself.

Varicose veins are a consequence of having a job you do not like or living in a place that does not suit you. Veins then lose their ability to be filled with joy.

The skin represents individuality. People with skin problems usually feel endangered and have a feeling that others rule over them. You have to accept yourself the way you are with all your strengths and flaws and you will be healed.

Arthritis is a disease caused by constantly criticizing yourself and others. Such people suffer from perfectionism and feel that they need to be perfect in every situation. It reflects the attitude that one does not consider oneself good enough and that one is difficult to live with.

People who perceive life as constant problem-solving do not have the feeling that life is love. In most life situations they get upset and see the potential for misfortune and tragedy in everything. Strokes, if they are less severe, usually force a person to think and move in a new direction and reevaluate their former way of life.

Homosexuality in men is a disease. The disease is defined in the mother's womb. Most food nowadays is filled with hormones. In most cases, female hormones are taken in order to improve the growth of animals that serve as food for humans. Since women in pregnancy consume such foods, there are hormonal changes in the baby. Later it manifests through male homosexual relationships.

In women, homosexuality is born out of great bitterness, disappointment and hurt, mostly by their male partners.

Allergies mostly develop in situations that are related to the environment. If the negative energy of annoyance and the hostility of people towards their environment are not resolved, they manifest in the physical body. In children, allergies develop because such energy is unconsciously transferred to them by their parents, or because they brought it with them in order to resolve a purpose in this physical life.

High cholesterol is the consequence of not accepting the joy of life. Relax and enjoy.

Snoring is a consequence of rejecting a change to old ways of thinking.

Cysts are clusters of deep distress.

Sciatica is a consequence of hypocrisy, fear of poverty, and fear of the future. In problems involving the lumbar part of the spine, there is usually rejection of accepting the work a person does. With people who have an extremely arched upper spine, there is a pronounced fear of poverty and loss of money, as well as a feeling that they have to do everything by themselves if they want to achieve or have something.

Back pain can occur due to the un-mourned death of a close person or due to rage towards someone close. The back is often a barometer for unexpressed feelings when people feel like they need support and courage to express themselves.

People who have thyroid problems feel humiliated. Everything they do, they have to achieve through hard work. They constantly have to fight for their rights and ideals, and they constantly think that it will never be their turn to relax. Goiters appear when people feel hate due to inflicted pain. They see themselves as victims. They feel that no matter how hard they try they will never make their plans a reality and this makes them feel unfulfilled.

Hemorrhoids occur due to fear of deadlines, a feeling of rage due to certain situations from the past, and fear of relief, as well as a fear of being burdened.

Gout is usually caused by a need for domination, impatience, and rage.

Gastritis occurs in people who for a long time cultivate insecurity. They feel as if they need to surrender to the faith, that they cannot affect any event occurring in their lives, and that they have to succumb to chaos.

Ulcers develop in people who think that they are not good enough. Such people constantly try to satisfy the needs of others. Their self-respect is minute. Furthermore, ulcers can develop due to repressed rage.

Kidney stones develop in people who carry within themselves accumulated, unresolved rage, whether it is related to their parent, guardian, business, or partner.

Low blood pressure is usually caused by the feeling of a lack of love in childhood, while with high pressure the causes are usually long-term unresolved emotional problems with colleagues from work, parents, guardians or a partner.

Tinnitus is a consequence of refusing to listen; such people are always at the center of attention. They do not accept their inner voice and are distinguished by their stubbornness.

Hip problems occur in people who have a feeling of fear carrying out of most of their decisions. They do not see real positive outcomes to their decisions, and it creates anxiety and uncertainty in them.

Insomnia is usually caused by fear, distrust of life, and a feeling of guilt.

Colds/viral infections are warnings that you cannot accept the state you are temporarily in. If someone makes you angry or you are worn out and would like a short vacation or some solace, your body reacts to your thoughts and brings you a situation to help you do what you intended. Regardless of the fact that most people are not aware of their thoughts the clever thing to do is to accept your body's reaction and get away from daily life for a couple of days. That way, you are letting your physical body know that you respect and appreciate it, that you listen to it and act in tandem with it in order to improve your entire body. During those couple of days, you enable your body to gather some energy and free itself from the accumulated tension that caused such a reaction in the first place (the cold/viral infection).

Glaucoma develops in people who do not forgive or ask for forgiveness; there is a feeling of pressure caused by the emotional harm that people drag along with them.

Anxiety develops through distrust towards life.

Suicide is an act based on complete separation from your selfhood. It is a complete misunderstanding of what a person really is at their core. It means completely ignoring love, utter alienation, and immense selfishness. People think that they will solve their problems in this way. They think that the next time will be easier and that their destiny will not be as hopeless. Those who do not believe in reincarnation think that they will end it now and that will be all there is to it. Since these people are very selfish, they are usually the ones who caused great problems for their families because they focused on themselves regardless of their empty phrases. Such people are very big-headed, are full of praise for themselves, and think that they are absolutely perfect and that nobody understands them because they are always right. Such people are egoists as well.

Suicide does not solve anything; one only does immense damage to oneself. Suicide says that a person is not worthy of life or love, so in this karmic world, causes and consequences have to start from the beginning.

If a parent or guardian has a self-destructive energy, they will unconsciously transfer that energy onto their child. The more you think about suicide, the more your children are in danger. The reactions to a child's life are, at the beginning, depression, lifelessness, and withdrawing into solitude. Later it develops into a more serious disease, a severe accident that can result in death, or suicide.

With milder forms of self-destruction, when a parent or a guardian is oriented towards the self and considers themselves to be a victim of their own life, reactions they experience to situations that happen to them also in a certain way appear in the life of their child, such as frequent troubles, wounds, accidents, frequent inflammations, insecurity, running away from the family environment, and later a possibility of more serious ailments in the physical body.

It is necessary for parents or guardians to change their pattern of thinking about their own self-destruction in order to help their child, because there are not many parents or guardians who are aware of their energetic influence on their child. Some, unfortunately, do not care, given their selfishness and egoism.

Some people claim that some magic or some other form of external negative force has struck them. Since you are what you believe, in most cases there is a belief that has been imposed on them by society. People who live in an environment that accepts such behavior as a normal – but not natural – occurrence in their society usually blame other people for every accident that happens to them. Considering their belief in the immense possibility of such occurrences, these kinds of people usually experience such situations. Due to these beliefs, a person can be struck by a serious ailment or die, but no signs of disease can be found during an autopsy. The negative energy of their belief in the negative abilities of another person causes such a powerful reaction in their bodies that they die.

There are situations when people blame another person for wanting them dead. Since they carry a pattern of self-destruction and also have read about such possibilities, they cause situations themselves because of negative energy in their energy field. They are so overwhelmed by it and are absolutely convinced that serious diseases, even death, occur without real cause.

It is therefore evident how enclosed people are in their physical world and how completely they are separated from God. People who are connected to God are absolutely protected from all negative influences and negative beliefs. They know that it is all an unreal and imaginary state of their environment. The correct state is living in love and peace and offering goodness to all people, animals, plants, and the Earth.

When you choose life in your mind, you have chosen for energy to flow through you. Death is the opposite choice when a person decides to move against the energy of life.

At every moment of their lives people are constantly confronting the choice between life and death, but they are not aware of it.

Every time a person chooses to believe in and follow their intuition, a channel through which they receive the energy of life widens and more life force flows through it. Body cells then receive more energy and regenerate faster. People then feel physically, emotionally, and mentally more alive, and their spiritual light is felt everywhere. The bodies of these kinds of people remain young, healthy, and beautiful, and they emanate vitality.

When people choose death, which means they do not follow their intuition, they close the channel of energy flow and their cells do not receive enough energy. The body then begins to fall apart rapidly. It will not always be evident in a person's appearance right away, but other people will feel very bad when they are near the person. When you do not follow the energy flow, life turns into a constant struggle. Stress and tension take their toll in the physical sense, and the struggle can then be visible on the physical body in the form of a disease. Moreover, due to constant troubles, the body begins arching forward under the burden of excessive struggles. If people change their relationship with themselves, so that they are more self-assured, their bodies start to regenerate.

One part always wants to live, to dedicate itself to life, and to believe in its intuition and follow it at every moment.

Whenever a person dies, they unconsciously choose to abandon their physical body. They can seem like victims of an accident or fatal disease, but it is not so. The Earth is a planet of free will, and everyone is the master of their own life's journey. The spirit knows what to do even if the physical body denies it.

Some people feel as though they are in a hopeless position and that nothing works as it should, so they believe that everything has conspired against them, and they unconsciously choose to end their lives in their physical bodies. However, if they realize that it is necessary to sail down the river of life with care, led by their intuition which is omniscient, they learn how to navigate through the occasional rapids, waterfalls, or narrow stony paths and enjoy this life. Going down the river leads to everything turning out in your favor, a life full of joy, as it in fact is.
Have faith and trust.

Listen to your body; it knows perfectly well what suits you, regardless of what it is: the food you consume, the color or piece of your clothes, the situation you are in, or the people you communicate with your body reacts to everything and sends signals to your consciousness.

The body is a basic feedback mechanism that shows what works in everyday thinking, expression, and living and what does not.

Most people, when it comes to their upbringing and their situation in life while they were children, do not have a natural attitude towards accepting and naturally solving problems that appear on our lives' paths. Such habits are created for people to survive in the chaotic world they live in. These habits are learned and accepted from parents, guardians, family, friends, and the community.

People imitate those around them and try to follow imposed rules, thereby turning against the flows of their own life energy. People then do not do what they actually feel within themselves. They stop paying attention to the signs sent by their bodies regarding food, rest, exercise, and the support they need. The constant repetition of certain actions starts to reflect on their physical body in the sense of arching forwards, as well as on the state of their spirit, so people let their environment know that they feel small and insignificant. Every time a person does not trust themselves and does not follow their inner truth, their vitality decreases, and their body loses its vitality and becomes dull, painful, and prone to diseases.

Our bodies are warning us in numerous ways, and it usually begins with a person feeling uncomfortable or becoming easily worn out. When this is not enough, the physical body will put in the effort to give a clearer warning, producing headaches, pain, and lesser ailments such as colds and viral infections. If a person does not notice it and does not react in the correct way by thinking about what causes such warnings, but simply takes a pill to ease the trouble, some more serious disease or accident can appear. Even in such cases, people still have the potential to alter their self-destructive attitudes and beliefs, and to heal; they just have to truly want to.

Once the physical body develops a symptom, it returns every time that person behaves in a similar way.

Accidents occur as a warning that people should not judge themselves or harm themselves within, and that they should let the feeling of guilt go, along with the need for self-punishment. Accidents are also a reflection of suppressed anger. They point to frustrations that make people want to confront the cause of their frustrations, but in the end, it comes back around to bite them.

There are situations in life that need to be respected. For example, a person sees a doctor for a physical examination, and they were healthy their entire life. It is determined that one kidney is almost invisible, which means that it has atrophied and ceased to function. The doctor advises urgent surgery so that the kidney does not damage the entire body. (In this situation the doctor does not know when the kidney started dying. Is it possible that the kidney has been in the body for years? Is it there and like that for a reason? The doctor also does not know the function of this kidney in relation to the entire body and the karmic pattern of the person in this life.) The surgery is scheduled; however, the surgeon has injured his hand and cannot operate. The operation is scheduled for later, but the surgeon falls ill. It clearly means that you are being warned against the surgery because that kidney is protecting you from serious health issues.

There are situations in which a tumor or any other serious disease breaks down in a short period of time and disappears without repercussions or coming back. Everything is possible through prayer. You need to realize that you have a risk of dying with any kind of surgery or any kind of thought-pattern that you have dealt with thus far. You need to make peace with the fact that everything you were attached to, or that you cherished most in life and that inspired secret aggression deep within you due to the possibility of it being lost, will disappear. Once you realize that, pray for the cleansing of your spirit before God. The aggression will then retreat, as well as the attachment, due to an understanding and acceptance of the self, and the disease will therefore be cured.

Everything that happens to you depends on your attitude towards people and your environment. If you think that you will gain weight after getting rid of some addiction, for instance smoking, your way of thinking will motivate your physical body, so it will very likely happen.

Laziness is a disease caused by sluggishness of emotions. Lazy people usually do not want to think about anything even when it is about themselves. They wait for others to do their personal and business chores and feel frustrated if they are forced to do something by themselves. They look for all possible means by which they can avoid any mental or physical work. It is usually their only amusement. When they think that they have achieved what they wanted, it makes them proud, which increases their ego. They are insensitive and important only to themselves. If they think that they will achieve something by fighting, they will do so until the other side surrenders. Behavior such as this lowers their energy, so they are prone to allergies and colds that look like they never cease.

Your inner, personal attitude towards yourself and how you see yourself in a certain situation defines how people around you will behave towards you.

One example is mobbing, or when you fear that you cannot express yourself, fear losing your job, fear that someone will misunderstand you, fear that you will do something wrong. Check where that feeling comes from. It is an unreal fear that damages not only you, but your environment as well since there is no natural communication. The same thing will keep happening to you until you realize that it stems from your childhood, when your parents or guardians told you that you will be nobody or that you are not trying hard enough because you will end up like them (poor). Poverty is a state of mind. Poor people are poor not only with respect to money but in emotions and in care and love as well, and they are separated from God, insecure and anxious.

Another example is abuse in the family circle. Usually, if one parent or guardian exacted physical violence on another, there is a strong possibility that the child, as an adult, will find a similar person as a partner. The similarity does not mean that the negative energy patterns in parents or guardians are the same as in the new relationship of now grown-up children. With parents or guardians, it can be jealousy or bitterness regarding their lives, while in the child who is now an adult; it is usually self-punishment to be with a person such as this, due to their parents' actions from their childhood.

A third example is a husband is cheating on his wife with another woman. In this case there is a strong combination of the roles of tyrant/victim. She feels like a victim, powerless, insecure, anxious, and hurt, and he, in doing this, wants to show himself how strong and all-powerful he is.

By understanding this situation and with the exchange of energies and a rise to the higher level (where positive energy is attracted through understanding), there is a complete change in the situation.

During conversations with other people, you are always mutually connected through the third and the fourth energy centers, that is, the solar plexus and the heart chakra (the energy center). When being close to or in conversation with certain people, you feel exhausted, while with others you feel excellent. People feel exhausted near people who possess a low level of energy and near people who are prone to diseases. It means that such people drain your energy. If you do not protect yourself from that, you will later need some time to recuperate from such conversations. Regardless of the fact that energies are not compatible and since every person has their frequency, such people can save themselves from a disease they are developing (which is most often the case). Such people are energy vampires. You can mostly recognize them by their fighting attitude. They constantly make excuses.

There is a situation in which a person willingly, but unconsciously, gives energy to someone from their family because they unconsciously feel that it will help their loved one to overcome an initial crisis.

You can protect yourself from the energy vampires using a simple exercise.

Imagine a cone impenetrable to any energy that could jeopardize you and put it around yourself. If you cannot visualize it (draw a mental picture), sketch it on a piece of paper. Put yourself inside the cone and feel excellent. Put another imaginary person without a first or last name on the other side. Or imagine that you are holding a shield (a knight's impenetrable shield) and nothing can touch you. Or ask God to protect you. He will gladly do it. You can do this before going to sleep, since your consciousness is most susceptible at that time, and because your physical body is relaxed, so your thoughts are as well. Asking God for help and protection can be done in any situation you are in. By frequently repeating a wish or request, you enter a stage of believing in help because your consciousness has completely accepted your wish. After some time, you will no longer need to pray; everything will be given to you as soon as you find yourself in such a situation.

Addictions develop when people need support and they have forgotten how to love themselves and are therefore running from themselves. This is when people begin smoking, taking drugs, and adopting other dangerous and unhealthy habits for their physical body. All addictions can be resolved, but it is necessary to take the first step and decide to do it. Later, simply ask for the strength to persist and withhold from your higher "self," but at the same time ask for faith in yourself and truth about what you truly in essence are. Such actions will cleanse you of the negative energy generated by your incorrect understanding of the self and your unhealthy emotions towards the self. Go to church often, but only when it is empty, so you can directly receive the positive energy you need. Accept it wholeheartedly and believe.

When you go to an empty church, it disables your negative energy you want to get rid of, that is to purify your body from mixing with other negative energies that exist when the church is filled with people. Since the energy fields of people constantly collide, whether by passing next to them, being near them, or talking to them, it is advisable that you turn to yourself to be alone with God as much as you can.

Do not pray for your children and grandchildren if you have not purified yourself first because then you can transfer their negative energy onto yourself or give yours to them. The more deeply you purify yourself, the more able you will be to help others. When you feel that nothing can affect your love towards God, regardless of the situation you are in, it means that you accept all obstacles that God gives you in your life as a means of learning and that you are capable of praying for others as well.

Temptation can be endured only by people who have the correct attitude towards life and are connected to their higher “self”. Life in its material sense should be observed as the constant loss of someone or something, at the end of which everything physically gained in life is lost in the sense of the individual values a person is attached to. From the spiritual side, life is a constant quest for love and truth and aspiration towards God. Therefore, we constantly win by understanding the numerous situations and events we go through in our lives.

The diseases that people are born with usually shock their parents or guardians because they occur regardless of a clear ultrasound and the fact that both parents are healthy. Such people choose this type of life on Earth in order to redeem themselves for some negative things that they watched from the sidelines or were directly included in during some of their previous lives. It is the simplest way for a soul to help itself in reducing its karmic purposes and lives. So, accept these people with love and help them to spend their lives in the best way that they can, in love.

Behave carefully towards everything. Everything you possess was made from someone's creative energy. If it were not for that person, you would not possess what you possess. Be careful and thankful for everything because you were allowed a quality life.

A small number of medical problems nowadays were caused by events from past lives. Since such events are exclusively related to unresolved feelings, it is possible to resolve them by dealing with those feelings in this physical life. Feelings as such do not change during time periods, only the thoughts causing various situations and events in order to experience a certain feeling; therefore, everything can be resolved, you just have to pray and believe.

Beliefs

People believe that every medicine they take will ease, alleviate, or completely cure their health issues. Over the centuries, the usage of various medications showed that, regardless of much new research and many findings over the past couple of decades, the rate of treatment success through the centuries is actually the same for some diseases. It is estimated that more than seventy percent of all forms of medical treatment have not been scientifically examined.

Research was conducted among groups of people who were told about the medicine they would be given and what kind of an effect it would have on their bodies. Then they were given a placebo. A placebo is the same shape as a pill but is sugar or a saline solution of distilled water with salt, which means that it does not have any effect on the human body. Half of the participants experienced the same effects as they would have if they had actually taken the real medicine. This shows that the human brain is keen on accepting the words that have been spoken, and it means that no medication is necessary in order to heal/cure the human body.

The opposite is true as well. If people take medicine – regardless of its ability to treat a certain medical condition – and are assured that it is not good for them, the medicine will not work at all, or will have the opposite effect.

Given the fact that every person is completely different in the way they think, accept new things, abandon old things, and hold on firmly their beliefs, every person needs a different amount of a certain medicine for it to work for their particular physical body. A doctor has to know if a person is often medicated or never takes any medication at all. Aspirin also counts as a medication. Under no circumstances should two completely different people take the same dosage of a particular medication because this worsens the body's energy structure with such differences that the effect on the physical body of a person who never takes pills and is defined as a healthy person is incredibly detrimental. It could manifest as vertigo, vomiting, or digestive issues.

Most people who are given a medication and who blindly trust their doctors do not read the warnings and side effects because if they did, all the pharmaceutical companies would go bankrupt. Medicines are taken at your own risk, since people are warned about possible contraindications and mostly there are warnings about how harmful a medication is for your body and what side effects might manifest on your other organs.

This only proves how much people trust their doctors when it comes to whether a recommended medication will help them.

If people read the warnings and see the side effects, they realize that they have to protect that other organ in some way. So, they buy a new medication that protects that other organ but see that it is insufficient because that medication affects some third organ and so on.

The way of understanding medications today and their use feeds and maintains the pharmaceutical industry, which is focused on maintaining only your physical body. Since the body is not only physical but energy as well, drugs suppress the real reason a person is feeling unwell – that the body's level of healing energy has decreased. People get sicker, have less energy, and look for an exit in the external world while running from themselves instead of looking for an answer within their bodies, where the answer is always located. It always is.

Medicine by itself lowers your energy because it forces you to suppress the feelings that caused pain or some change in your body. You do not let yourself communicate with your own body; you try to hush everything up. It causes your physical body to suffer and age, to feel misunderstood and painful. The physical body is then forcefully closed off to possible self-healing and prosperity.

People are deeply attached to their beliefs. If they have bad eyesight, they believe it is permanent and that it will worsen. Nobody thinks that the disease will go away by changing their mood or way of thinking. Thoughts can manage all things, including your body's health. Simple and ordinary belief can have a strong effect on the body. Since most people do not possess mental discipline, they cannot manage their beliefs. In order for people to gain control, they first have to understand the various forms of the beliefs that affect them because they offer a view on the relationship of positive energy of thought and the physical body.

Cultural beliefs are beliefs forced upon a person by society: the belief that a girl who is not married by a certain age will remain a spinster all her life, which means that she will never marry or the belief that clothes make the man, and when a person starts talking, it would have been better if they had not.

Cultural beliefs are connected to behavior and mutual relationships in society, their fears, and the ways we react to them. This develops negative patterns of thinking and behavior that enter the energy fields of individuals who live in a certain area and are linguistically or religiously connected. Such negative energy fields cause the same or similar anomalies in the physical body, so we say that there are more people suffering from heart disease in some places, and in some others there are more diabetics, and in the next one alcoholic. If people do not understand the energy pattern that is at work in their environment, they are completely or partially susceptible to those energies because of their way of thinking. Through a stronger cleansing of bodily energy, by raising your body to a higher positive energy level, the body is less susceptible to external influences because it works as a natural defense mechanism. The purer the body is, the less it is susceptible to external influences.

Beliefs are embodied by attitudes. In attitudes and diseased states of the body, a fighting spirit could be highlighted as the strongest. With people who suffer from so-called serious, incurable diseases, it has been shown that a fighting spirit affects the length of their lives. When people give up, they die immediately. The attitudes of a pregnant woman towards her child determine whether there will be complications in pregnancy or during childbirth, as well as what health issues the child will have after its birth. If her attitude is positive, the positive energy she has towards her pregnancy and child will protect her and her child from negative external influences, negative energies from her environment, and the negative attitudes of the people surrounding her.

Beliefs expressed through the strength of their own will are considered passive beliefs, imposed on people by their culture or common thinking. If people are convinced that they can help themselves using their abilities and willingly managing the biological processes of the body, they can truly help themselves. In order to achieve this, discipline is necessary, as well as faith and a positive mindset. With their attitudes and way of thinking, people can go through fire without getting burned or can lift immensely heavy objects without experiencing any consequences in their physical body afterwards. Everyone can willingly learn to manage their body, and in such a way, take responsibility for their own health.

Unconscious beliefs affect changes in behavior and changes in the energy structure of the body. Since people are not aware of them, hypnotherapists and psychotherapists can be of great help in such situations. Hypnotherapy is established in some countries, while in others it is still being developed. In the countries where it is developed, it is possible to ask for adequate help and you will receive it, and in the others, one should be very careful. When you see doctors of hypnotherapy, it is necessary for them to be academically educated, unbiased, completely healthy mentally, able to understand the self in order to understand the person who will be treated with hypnosis, and a patient should have immense trust in them. The reason for this is that hypnotherapists mostly do deep hypnosis, which means that the physical body is not aware of the situation it is in. A hypnotherapist enters into the patient's unconscious, and if he is not a good doctor, he can cause more harm than good. He searches your unconscious for events that caused certain reactions and emotions in your body that manifested in your physical body as diseases. The things that have happened to you happened for a reason. In order to protect themselves, people repress these things, so a doctor of hypnotherapy will try to reveal what was buried deep down. He has to explain everything after the therapy and talk you through it in order for you to understand and accept and forgive yourself and others if it was caused by a certain event.

Since patients are unaware of everything, and since the doctor is in a position of power over your unconscious which is receptive to absolutely all suggestions when it is in this state, if he is not a professional, he can cause even bigger problems. He can suggest that you do something that will, according to him, help you but which can be completely unacceptable for your soul's growth, or he can erase some events, so patients feel certain emptiness, as if something is missing, which prevents people from realizing and resolving one or more of the medical problems they have.

A good hypnotherapist can cure absolutely all diseases because positive suggestion initiates a stream of consciousness opposite to one that was placed in your energy field. If you are convinced that some disease is incurable because you were told so or convinced, then only suggestion under deep hypnosis can lead to complete healing in a short period of time by making you better each day and making your body heal and the disease disappear. This means that the disease will not return in any form.

Patients have the ability to participate in light trance hypnosis because they enter a lower level of unconsciousness through this therapy. With such forms of therapy, patients are in a deep state of relaxation, almost a stupor, which should not worry anyone, since one movement of a toe can return the body into its former state. Patients participate by responding to the doctor's questions, by seeing pictures or films, sensing smells, or feeling a touch through their inner eye in order to realize what happened in those unresolved and misunderstood situations in a completely unbiased way. It is the most natural form of hypnotherapy and it is the best for most patients. Deep hypnotherapy is better for people who have unreasonable fears.

A psychotherapist must have a deep knowledge of human emotions in order to help people understand the relationship between feelings and the development of certain health disorders.

Beliefs embodied in faith refer to people who believe that, if they visit a place sacred to their religion, it will enable them to heal. This happens very often, and it all depends on the strength of one's faith. The first reaction to healing is always pleasant warmth. There are situations when a person loses a part of a bone or a part of the body due to a disease, which regenerates completely after visiting a sanctuary. Bone regeneration was mentioned simply because it is a very rare occurrence.

All cells possess a mind, which means that they know perfectly well what function they have, and when one dies, they know how another one should be created in order for the physical body to function well, so with this procedure, the entire process is accelerated.

Belief that you will get help once you have arrived at some sanctuary is reinforced by the fact that such places have a high concentration of positive energy.

Such belief in your body includes taking in a lot of positive energy towards yourself, showing selfless love towards the self, so such love heals with its strength. Love is an all-powerful, limitless positive energy that heals all events, emotions, and the entire physical body. In love, a person is completely healthy.

There is a belief that an addiction to caffeine and nicotine, as well as drugs, can exist; this is incorrect. Research was conducted and there was proof that nothing can affect the physical body if it was not defined so in one's pattern of belief. Belief forced upon a person by society is emphasized. Caffeine does not wake you up, nor does nicotine relax you, but by lowering your energy, you become more nervous, insecure, and anxious over time.

There are no incurable diseases; everything is within one's patterns of belief.

Purity of intention is very important in the desire to heal. It will direct you correctly. You will feel some of the ways that could help you get rid of the disease within yourself perfectly clearly. Your intuition will lead you to the best possible way to solve a problem. With some problems, a close person will be enough, while with other problems you will ask for a doctor's advice or solve the problem in a sanctuary. The answer is always within you, so get connected to yourself and get rid of the disease.

Your body possesses all of God's powers, which are waiting for you to call on them and use them. You are here to reveal how competent, sublime, and noble you are. You are here to live a full and happy life in harmony with your mission on Earth, in harmony with the Universe and God.

Discard old beliefs that lead you to situations that do not suit you. Discard those conclusions of your negative thoughts and emotions that tell you that you have to suffer, be poor, and unsuccessful. Get out of the rut; free yourself from the patterns created in childhood, as well as of unhealthy habits concerning your diet, behavior and way of living. Stop repeating patterns of behavior forced upon you by your society, culture, or religion. Stop thinking that everything you were told contains the truth of living within itself. Millions of people nowadays cherish ancient, meaningless, and regressive beliefs about the laws of life, although many know that they are wrong and laughable. Let truth and God's love enter your life and your way of thinking, behaving, and feeling, so you can become what you are, an absolutely healthy person filled with God's love.

The universal life principle, our intuition, is constantly trying to express itself through us when we are open to it. By connecting yourself with your heart, you receive ideas that enable you to improve your situation in life. Desires, aspirations, urges, and the deepest drives of your heart can reach God. Accept them and sense how well you feel with those thoughts. If you feel well, calm, and at the same time exhilarated, go through it with your entire heart and all the positive energy will help you to realize it in the most positive way for you and your environment.

In unity with God you are protected from all negative energies from the external world and you accept Godly virtues: harmony, peace, inspiration, leadership, and God's righteous actions. You will then realize that your thoughts are calm, irrespective of the situation, and that you are growing as a person if you are ready to accept positive energy and live in it and with it.

In medical circles, it is a well-known fact that people in moments of great fear, immediate danger, shock, and tragedy do marvelous things. Disabled people walk, and the paralyzed are cured. People in such moments have an incredible wish to save their lives or the lives of their loved ones under any circumstances. From a positive attitude come positive healing and the liberating energy of love, which can do absolutely anything. It shows that such power exists in you from the moment you are born, but you have not used it before now.

God never avenges nor punishes. We are all thinkers, responsible for our way of thinking. Therefore, every person is unique. You have the power to choose. If you opt for prayer and meditation, you are moving in a positive direction towards your goal.

People are given free will at birth and are determined by it. Since God is only an observer who will gladly jump in and help if you ask Him, He will, through certain events, strive to direct you towards the correct path, but He will never force you to do anything or punish you if you did not understand His intentions. It is a good enough reason to open your eyes and ears and observe, conclude, and connect in order to understand. He is always there for you and because of you, and if you need or ask something, He will always lend you a hand, no matter how strange, inconvenient or sometimes unacceptable it may look from your point of view. It is all a matter of the attitude that you have towards things, and everything should be observed from a point of learning and direction towards your selfhood because God does exactly that.

Millions of people refuse to hear the truth. They do not comprehend, and many refuse to accept the fact that each man is his own savior, shaping and creating his own destiny. They refuse to accept the truth that they have to assume responsibility for their own actions.

Millions of people are lazy and negligent nowadays. They carry all of God's power within themselves, but rarely, if at all, look for that power and use it. God does not make differences between people. God's law is equal for all people. God will grant even the prayers of an atheist, of someone who claims that God does not exist. No one can stand between you and God. You do not need sermons and ceremonies. You do not need to belong to any organization nor religion. When you address God's presence, it will reply. You do not need intermediaries, only your own thoughts. Your thoughts are a mediator between the visible and invisible, and if you continue to ponder eternal truths, you will experience a holiness that represents perfect health, harmony, and peace, and you will have all the riches you need to live in peace and harmony and not be burdened by anything.

However insensible and mistaken you are, you can at any moment address God's providence, and you will get help immediately. God is timeless and space-less.

Every problem that you carry with you carries within itself an overwhelming desire to be solved. So, turn your back on worldly external searching for a solution to your problems, and turn to your inner power because God's power and wisdom will always be with you. Be adamant in that belief and your problems will disperse in the light of God's love.

The power within us is ready to help us realize our craziest dreams and our immense potential. The problem is that most people, since they do not realize or accept this, are not open to receiving it. For most people, such a thought is frightening because they think that opening themselves up would mean receiving terrifying things, which is probably true since their pattern of behavior is directed towards this.

The law of cause and effect works on all levels. If we take from others, we lose. If we give, we gain. It cannot be any other way. If people disparage or judge others, they will be judged as well. If people are always angry, they meet anger wherever they go. The love people have towards themselves is in harmony with love that life feels towards those people. If they have taken something from somebody, and afterwards lost something, it is necessary for them to realize the connection between these two experiences.

There is a connection on different levels. For example, when people take something that does not belong to them, they almost always lose something more valuable. They can take money or some item and lose a valuable relationship. If they steal a relationship from someone, they could lose a job. If they steal a pen or something similar from the office, they can be late for their commute or an important dinner. Such loss always hurt people in a very significant area of their lives.

If you have suffered a lot of loss in your life or many things have gone wrong, it would be good to question the way you take things.

Even people who would never consider stealing something steal other people's time and self-respect.

Every time another person feels guilty because of your words or behavior, you steal their self-worth.

Being truly fair on all levels requires great reassessment and full awareness.

When people take something that does not belong to them, they actually inform the all-knowing and ever-present positive energy that they are unworthy of earning money by themselves, that they are not good enough, and that they want to be stolen from because they are unworthy of possessing something. Some think that they have to be mean and cunning in order to possess something, but such an opinion blurs their vision and prevents them from experiencing abundance and joy in life.

This planet is wealthy. Good always comes to us in harmony with our conscience. Being absolutely fair is a choice a person has to make out of love towards themselves. Living fairly ensures an easier and more comfortable life. If you do not get charged for something at the store, your moral obligation, if you have noticed it, is to say something.

Everything that surrounds you is a reflection of what you believe you deserve. Look at your home. Does it suit you; is it comfortable; do you feel peace and serenity while you are in it? Does it exude love? The clothes you wear are a reflection of what you feel about yourself, and the color of the clothes you wear is a reflection of your attitude towards yourself.

Personal relationships are the most important for most people. People always seek love. When people do not find the romantic partner they want, it means that they have not defined well what exactly they expect from that person, so the reason for love is unclear. There is a large difference between the need for love and the hunger for love. The hunger for love is a need for love towards the self. People then enter relationships in which they are dependent, and this is inefficient for both partners. Such a relationship is sought in order for a person to feel fulfilled beside another person. If you tell another person what to do, then you manipulate the relationship. Think about your negative beliefs from childhood that are now having an impact on your relationship, which should be positive for both parties. Define new positive beliefs and stick to them no matter how many times you unconsciously return to the old ones.

A large number of people would rather everyone else around them change, rather than changing themselves. This refers to everyone in their family, at work, those who have an impact on changes in their environment and, indirectly, everything else that is related to them in some way. The only possibility for change is within that person themselves. If you want to improve your life, change is essential. So, changes within should start slowly and gradually. If you change only a bit, you will feel better. Such change will motivate you to make further changes. Later, when you develop a rhythm, everything will seem smooth and simple.

Inner change is simple; you just need to kick-start it with a decision because all you need to change are your thoughts. You can get help in numerous ways: by receiving a book, through new acquaintances or new events, a new job, or a new partner.

By working on yourself, you help in raising the positive energy of, not only your environment, but of the Earth as well.

Cloning, Transplants and Transfusions

Cloning

When scientists began researching the possibilities of creating new living organisms from a single cell, they created a sheep, which came as a revolutionary discovery. It meant that two individuals defined by the basic laws of life, a male and a female, were not needed to create a living organism. This discovery launched an avalanche of outcry, of course, for a good reason. Scientists did not think about the negative consequences of their negative creations but only about satisfying their own egos. It is known that, over time, situations simmer down, so they knew that people's unconscious minds would react, regardless of their refusal to accept, in order to make peace with a situation they cannot change anyway. At this time, they were doing research on people, and they offered women, mostly businesswomen, the chance to create a child without having to go through pregnancy, and there they found fertile ground since those women think egotistically in the same way that they do.

In the meantime, scientists began toying with the mutation of various plant cells, all with the idea of improving life and improving the quality of plants and their resistance to various pests. The fact that various pests appear has always been true and always will be, so there will be enough food for humans after them and with them. Scientists do not care about this; they care only about creating something, regardless of whether it creates large-scale cell mutations in humans who have to adapt to a new diet. The cycle on Earth that was created by God has its reasons, and it needs to be respected and adapted to because otherwise everything disintegrates and disappears. It has always been so. It is evident that, the more developed the civilization, the more damage it does to living organisms on Earth. The reason for this is that scientists, oriented towards creating living organisms from cells, have completely lost their connection to God. They are playing with something they do not understand. They become wanton and negligent towards the life happening around them. They have lost their knowledge about the true laws of life.

Civilizations that are considered backward are happier, more satisfied, and more open to receiving goodness and love into their hearts. They do not even think about disturbing God's order. They sense that it could completely destroy life in their environment so they often pray for guidance and answers to the question of whether something can be done or not. Their lives consist of conversation and unity with God, the creator of all that is visible and invisible. Therefore, their lives are careless and healthy.

Scientists have lost their connection to God, and given their growing egos, it is unlikely – although absolutely possible – that they will reach the understanding that nothing that is not in harmony with God will survive.

Since cloning is performed by extracting DNA from a cell's nucleus and placing it in the egg of a woman, such an organism has no soul. A soul is given by God during natural conception. People created from such embryos walk the Earth like zombies, soulless people so different that they need to be fed. Producing such people creates overcrowding on the already overcrowded Earth, and at the same time, an increase in famine. That means that food production would need to be significantly increased.

Scientists have taken another step, telling those people, who think that they cannot solve their problems through their faith in God, that they can keep those clones since their organs have the same cellular structure as the DNA placed in a woman's egg, and that their clone will, should they have need of transplant, donate them a perfect organ. It would mean the conscious killing of a clone in order to satisfy the lowest of human needs. These are the lowest needs because those people who would demand such things have completely lost their connection to themselves, and they seek all their solutions in the external world.

By cloning animals, scientists want to achieve bigger alimentary possibilities for people. However, since an animal created in this way has no energy value, when consuming such meat, there is a complicated genetic mutation in the body of a person who eats it. Instead of guiding them towards the light and the purification of the physical body, it leads a person's body into becoming denser, into an even greater separation from the self.

God created plants that contain incredibly high amounts of energy. This energy is necessary for the organism to develop; it is not for the pure consumption of physical plants. Various mutations made by scientists make plants lose the essence for which they were created by God. Mutations lower the level of energy in a plant, either by hybridizing incompatible plant cells, by hybridizing cells with poisons that affect various pests in order for the plant to become resistant, or by hybridizing it with drugs. In any case, a certain level of negative energy occurs, which when it enters the organism, leads to cell mutation and to illness. The essence of a plant is thereby decreased because it does not contain a high concentration of positive energy that is necessary as food for the physical body.

This is the way to create even more imbalance on Earth.

Scientists do not understand that a human's purpose on Earth is the growth of their soul and not keeping the physical body alive. Since the clones that they create have no soul, they cannot consciously communicate or be naturally included in life. They are completely dependent on others. They are the image of the person from whom they have received their DNA. They grow the same and develop the same. Life without a soul has no sense of purpose. Scientists and people like them do not understand that the purpose of life is birth, life, ennobling the soul during one's life, and dying in a physical body. Therefore, the soul is what is, has always been, and will always remain until the end of times.

This way of thinking will completely disappear when people realize that the soul is eternal and that they have entered into a human body and live in it exclusively because of their soul. The only thing that matters is that after learning and living through the purpose that it was given in the physical world, the soul returns to eternal light and eternal love because it came from there.

Transplants and Transfusions

Using organs that have been grown in clones is less dangerous than using organs from other living or dead organisms. Every organ has its own genetic structure, and by placing such organs into their body, the patient who is determined to extend their lifespan in an artificial and unnatural way, is in fact putting themselves in an unenviable position. By receiving the organs of others, he transfers not only the genetic aspect but also the energy that organ possesses.

Given the energy that the organ carries, which is from a living donor, the patient also absorbs the energy of that individual, which means that his energy and the energy of the donor are constantly intertwining. Along with the organ's energy, the patient is also given the donor's patterns of behavior, which he must resolve along with his own. In addition, if the donor dies before the patient, that individual's energy remains in the patient, meaning a part of the donor's soul. The donor cannot leave; they are forced to remain on Earth along with the patient until the patient dies.

All organs have a certain frequency. The donor's organ, therefore, has a different frequency to that of the patient's body, the organ's recipient. Given that doctors do not understand this kind of connection, donor's organs that do not have a similar frequency to that of the patient are inevitably rejected.

For those individuals who have received organs from donors more than once, their lives become ever more complicated. Patients always feel the presence of the other energy in a particular way and at all times, and they cannot free themselves of it. This frequently leads to discomfort and insecurity, irrespective of the noble intentions of the donor.

This situation has appeared only because people are, more and more, detaching from their very selves, from unity with God. They see their bodies as exclusively physical, where the soul is just a secondary phenomenon. The physical body on its own does not possess a particularly significant meaning, but by ascribing it ever-greater meaning, people begin to orient themselves towards it and lose the real sense and reason for their presence on Earth. Given that they are oriented towards the physical, they are terrified of death and the loss of the physical with which they have identified, and they search for various means by which they might improve that physical body and extend its life.

A more complex problem appears with transfusions than with transplants because blood, the source of physical life, mixes directly the genetic DNA structures of donors and patients.

DNA structures contain a karmic pattern, which mean that every physical body, at the moment of its birth, receives an energy pattern it must purify throughout its life through its comprehension and understanding of the reasons that it entered into a physical body. In this way, the patient receives the donor's karmic structure alongside its own. This resembles the way that two people, two spirits, live in one physical body because the patient's physical body has two energy patterns. Given that energy is boundless, in every living and non-living creature, the energy of the donor is not divided, nor does it decrease.

In the case of two spirits in one physical body, the patient must also clear out the donor's patterns of behavior without even being aware of this. Situations will arise that never occurred to him or which did not occur under similar conditions, and he will not be able to connect them with anything. In addition, if he does not resolve the donor's energy patterns in this life, he will need to resolve them in one of his next lives, given that the Earth is based upon the law of cause and effect. Transfusions are very problematic for childbearing women and women who have yet to become mothers because they transfer the donor's energy pattern to their children.

The physical body's purpose is to carry the soul, and the purpose of the soul is to develop within the physical body through various events and situations. If you wish to extend your life in your physical body, it is only necessary to live in keeping with and as one with God.

An Interpretation of the Book of Genesis

Given that man is oriented towards the physical body, the material, the Book of Genesis is written in the same manner. But:

The First Day
"In the beginning, when God created the heavens and the earth—and the earth was without form or shape, with darkness over the abyss and a mighty wind sweeping over the waters—Then God said: Let there be light, and there was light. God saw that the light was good. God then separated the light from the darkness. God called the light "day," and the darkness he called "night." Evening came, and morning followed—the first day."

One is the number of the creator, God himself. This is the first vibration of creation. Thus, then consciousness spread, God's ever-present light. The energy of consciousness was created by the omniscient and omnipresent light that allowed all things including the darkness; this is God. Consciousness, the creator of all worlds, allowed movement, which means the permeation of creative energy through everything that was created in the beginning. After this, thought was created as an expression of consciousness through which the vibrational interconnection of everything was made possible. (Thought is a vibration that does not disappear but develops). The light that is identified as an appearance of this first day of the Creation likewise emerged from a projection of the consciousness, the primary movement through which the entire Universe was created.

The Second Day

The words female and male are archaic terms of the whole of existence on Earth. This has nothing to do with gender.

"Then God said: Let there be a dome in the middle of the waters, to separate one body of water from the other. God made the dome, and it separated the water below the dome from the water above the dome. And so it happened. God called the dome "sky." Evening came, and morning followed—the second day."

The Second Day of Creation determines the division of the whole, the separation of all of Creation into two equal halves, the polarization of consciousness into two complementary aspects. Thus, an eternal attraction and repulsion was created, a movement of energy. From the moment of the division of God's whole, opposite poles long for union and to converge once more into a single whole, and this is the dynamic tension that makes up the whole of material reality. This is defined as electromagnetic dynamics, the symbol of male-female polarity.

The Third Day

"Then God said: Let the water under the sky be gathered into a single basin, so that the dry land may appear. And so it happened: the water under the sky was gathered into its basin, and the dry land appeared. God called the dry land "earth," and the basin of water he called "sea." God saw that it was good. Then God said: Let the earth bring forth vegetation: every kind of plant that bears seed and every kind of fruit tree on earth that bears fruit with its seed in it. And so it happened: the earth brought forth vegetation: every kind of plant that bears seed and every kind of fruit tree that bears fruit with its seed in it. God saw that it was good. Evening came, and morning followed—the third day."

The Third Day of the Book of Genesis brings with it three elements: the dry earth as a new aspect of existence, the sky, and the sea. These three elements symbolize the Holy Trinity. This is the father, mother, and child, the sperm, egg, and fetus. This is the unspeakably powerfully depicted power of the creativity of life experiences. This meaning comes from polarity and resolves the division of the whole.

It is necessary to understand that vibration is the attraction of electricity (active consciousness) and its polar aspect, magnetism (unconscious receptivity). The Earth symbolizes the crystallization of the interactivity between electricity and magnetism into being, which means the appearance of a new form – life.

The Fourth Day

"Then God said: Let there be lights in the dome of the sky, to separate day from night. Let them mark the seasons, the days and the years, and serve as lights in the dome of the sky, to illuminate the earth. And so it happened: God made the two great lights, the greater one to govern the day, and the lesser one to govern the night, and the stars. God set them in the dome of the sky, to illuminate the earth, to govern the day and the night, and to separate the light from the darkness. God saw that it was good. Evening came, and morning followed—the fourth day."

The fourth day represents knowledge of the cycle of the nature of life in physical reality. The natural cycle of life on Earth is determined by the Sun and Moon, described as two lights. The Sun, as the larger light, becomes the central point around which the Earth moves, while the Moon, the smaller light, has an orbit around the Earth. If the previous model of the lifecycle is followed, the Sun becomes the primary driver of life on Earth just as the Earth is to the Moon. Everything in the entire Universe is defined in this way, as is reflected from subatomic particles through cells to the construction of bodies.

The next part describes the appearance of the Sun and the Moon's lights, which regulate night and day and define the rotation of the Earth on its axis. Four seasons mark the full rotation of the Earth around the Sun and the way of measuring time using a calendar, while the Moon's four phases mark one full rotation of the Moon around the Earth.

Four defines the four elements: earth, air, fire and water on the Earth; the four directions of movement: forwards and backwards, left and right; the four seasons: spring, summer, autumn and winter, the Earth's rotation around the Sun; the Moon's four phases: new moon, first quarter, full Moon, and the last quarter. Everywhere there is stability and order.

The fourth day of the Book of Genesis is related to the force behind the natural cycles of the nature of life; it defines the rhythm of the Earth and the sharing of God's all-creating consciousness on the physical level, physical reincarnation.

The Fifth Day

"Then God said: Let the waters teem with abundance of living creatures, and on the earth let birds fly beneath the dome of the sky. God created the great sea monsters and all kinds of crawling living creatures with which the waters teem, and all kinds of winged birds.

God saw that it was good, and God blessed them, saying: Be fertile, multiply, and fill the water of the seas; and let the birds multiply on the earth. Evening came, and morning followed—the fifth day."

Five numerically represents the pentagon and its inner pentagram (a star with five points), which is the predominant geometric form in all living creatures and which manifests in the body of many animals and people. It represents life-force, consciousness, which breathes life into the elements in harmony with all living things. This represents God's voice (conscious desire), which activated the process.

The Sixth Day

"Then God said: Let the earth bring forth every kind of living creature: tame animals, crawling things, and every kind of wild animal. And so it happened: God made every kind of wild animal, every kind of tame animal, and every kind of thing that crawls on the ground. God saw that it was good. Then God said: Let us make human beings in our image, after our likeness. Let them have dominion over the fish of the sea, the birds of the air, the tame animals, all the wild animals, and all the creatures that crawl on the earth. God created mankind in his image; in the image of God he created them; male and female he created them. God blessed them and God said to them: Be fertile and multiply; fill the earth and subdue it. Have dominion over the fish of the sea, the birds of the air, and all the living things that crawl on the earth. God also said: See, I give you every seed-bearing plant on all the earth and every tree that has seed-bearing fruit on it to be your food; and to all the wild animals, all the birds of the air, and all the living creatures that crawl on the earth, I give all the green plants for food. And so it happened. God looked at everything he had made and found it very good. Evening came, and morning followed—the sixth day."

In this section, one can note that God defines Himself as "us" and man as "them". This reflects an understanding of consciousness that all thoughts are waves that permeate everything, that is, everything that exists, recognizing themselves as an endless vibration and frequency.

The majority of people believe in the figure of the Father as the human form because of the term "in His image", but God is everywhere. He is total consciousness, and He encompasses and permeates everything seen and unseen. God represents the macro-universe, while man represents the micro-universe, which means that everything is created from the same and everything is the same.

The definition of the creation of male and female is not defined in the common understanding of gender but in the sense that everything is as one and contains elements of yang (male) and yin (female) energy as man (the manifestation of consciousness). Every human being is conceived of as yang-yin, male-female, an electromagnetic union of consciousnesses.

The macro/micro Universe that follows the meaning of "fill the earth" should be understood in the sense of spreading the light of consciousness, and "subdue it" represents the enlightenment of your lower "I" (the ego) and an enlightened life (a higher self) in which the goal of the micro-universe is to return to the macro-universe, that is, for man to return to God.

The domination of man over all living things is God's request to man that he raise himself up above other creatures and completes the purpose for which he has been placed on Earth, which is to bring light to all the cellular structures of everything that exists on Earth.

On the sixth day, man is given a blessing to become a light-bearing being, a being of light. This explains to man why he should not eat meat (given that meat makes him a denser being) but rather that he feed himself only with seed-bearing plants because they are full of light and cleanse man's dense body, thus meeting man's need to cleanse himself and God's reason for creating man on Earth: that he may become a light-bearing being. (Every physical body is made up of dense, materialized energy.)

The Seventh Day

"Thus the heavens and the earth and their entire array were completed. On the seventh day God completed the work he had been doing; he rested on the seventh day from all the work he had undertaken. God blessed the seventh day and made it holy, because on it he rested from all the work he had done in creation."

Seven represents the seven directions, the seven days of the week, the seven energy centers, the seven colors of the rainbow, the seven notes in a musical scale and numerous other systems. This is a spectrum, a prism, and a sound: levels, wrappers, and shapes. The seventh is a holy day of rest for many religious and traditions.

Seven belongs to the creation of colors, music and spirituality that emerge from divine creativity that determines and defines all things that create harmony between sounds, colors, and souls.

On the seventh day, God created divine harmony amongst everything that had been created in the first six days and aligned it with the souls of all living things on Earth.

Given that everything in creation has energy, this means that everything within us and outside of us is energy; we are all interconnected with everything else. This means that every being is connected to all the people on Earth, all the animals, the plants and with the Earth, and with everything in the Universe.

Everything is energy, everything is one consciousness, everything is completely connected, and everything is one in God.

PART IV

Part I
Ending Relationships, Attachments and Connections

This is a technique via which you can end unhealthy relationships and connections and transform them into natural, that is healthy, relationships in the most painless, acceptable, and positive way.

The earliest attachments are formed during childhood, and are formed with parents, guardians, close relatives, brothers and sisters, teachers, friends, and all those who have an impact on a child in any way, or who program them. Later attachments are established with friends, lovers, marriage partners, other members of one's family, children, or with those people to whom the individual turns to in search of security, whether they be alive or dead. There are other subtle relationships as well, for example, a relationship created by the wish that things are always the way that we want them to be, or we become attached to our ideas or to powerful emotions such as anger, jealousy, fear or pride. Relationships can also be created by the desire for things such as food, alcohol, drugs, money, gold, clothing, shoes, houses, cars, power, social status, education, or success, which are just some examples out of many.

An attachment to one's own physical life creates in human beings an intense fear of death.

Any act of rejection, whether the person responsible for it is aware of it or not, has a negative impact on the behavior of the rejected individual. We all know that there are parents who desperately wish for a child of a particular gender, and when they are disappointed, act very emotionally when the child is not of that gender. The baby experiences this reaction as a rejection, and this will affect them throughout their life because their entry into this world is tied to insecurity and rejection by the two people who should have offered them their very first sense of security. Rejection early on, even when the parent begins to love the child with time, creates the conditions for a range of negative reactions towards life. Some people will constantly search for situations in which they will be rejected because it is a condition that is familiar to them, and they therefore feel, in a strange way, secure. Others go through life constantly searching for love and attention in order to quench their thirst for acceptance, but they are never satisfied, no matter how much they receive.

Apart from an unwanted gender, a parent can, at the moment of their child's birth or in their early childhood, distance themselves from the child for other reasons as well. Some parents are upset if their child is not that beautiful when it is born, or if it does not develop as quickly as other children of the same age, particularly the children of relatives or friends, among whom there is frequently ruthless competition. Whatever the reason, rejection will create suffering and sorrow in the future.

Sometimes rejection cannot be avoided. For example, parents or guardians cannot avoid their fate when a child loses one or both parents or guardians at an early age, and the child's mind is not yet developed enough for the loss to be explained and correctly understood. Given that the child continues to understand such a loss as a rejection, the adult must confront this should they wish to free themselves from its consequences and consciously change their ideas.

Sometimes it seems that a rejection is too insignificant to cause problems in the future. It is the manner in which the child reacts to the situation, not the severity of the act of rejection itself that determines its impact on their behavior and conduct as an adult.

Carl Gustav Jung offered the world a theory that suggested that in every man, there is a female aspect called the anima and that in every woman, there is a male aspect that he called the animus.

The patterns of these aspects are predetermined based on how an individual reacts to examples of the masculinity or femininity of their parents. As these patterns develop unconsciously, people are not always aware of the process and believe that when they choose partners they are acting as free individuals.

In every man, given that he has male and female aspects, it would be natural that his male aspect dominates and that the female aspect merely supports him. For women, it would of course be natural for her female aspect to dominate and for the male to support it. The balance can be thrown off in countless ways, depending on the way the individual reacted to their parents' attitude to their own gender. In addition, the individual is born with a particular energy pattern, which contains the inherited propensities of their parents or guardians and inheritances from their previous lives. We have all met men who have very little connection with their female aspect and therefore lack the capacity for emotion. Women who are very feminine do not have sufficient contact with their male aspect and lack the ability to think clearly.

When people love one another, it would be natural for individuals who enter into a life together to help each other so that they might both create a better balance in their lives and raise your energies. (This means men and women; in other kinds of relationships they cannot be helped together and individuals in such relationships must be helped separately.) Each of the partners needs to work on reducing their excessively developed functions or characteristics within themselves in order to create their own personal balance; they should not rely on each other because in doing so, they become more connected instead of freeing themselves and living in a healthy partnership. If they manage to help each other in a mutual way, a healthy and dynamic union forms in which the partners will help each other on the path towards personal completeness and not mutual dependence. If they achieve this before one of them dies, it will be much easier for them to deal with the separation and adapt to their new life. Many of them are not prepared to change and will struggle against every change.

Parents and guardians should release their children from their influence after the age of twelve. Irrespective of this, parents and guardians remain figures of authority up until the time when the child begins developing its own independence and grows up.

It is important that the parent or guardian ends their relationship with a child that has died, irrespective of the child's age, in order to release the child, after its death, of earthly life and in order to shorten the mourning period.

The breaking of the connection is also recommended in cases of both deliberate and spontaneous pregnancy terminations. Miscarriages are usually accompanied by great sadness on the part of the parents, who awaited the birth of their child with joy. The mother also suffers because her bodily rhythm is thrown off, and she requires help with this as well. Mothers frequently blame themselves in the case of miscarriages, thinking they did something wrong. This is a way in which they can free themselves of the guilt that they feel, which weighs on them, and they can search for forgiveness from the soul that did not have the chance to enter into a physical body.

When it comes to abortions, there is a conscious decision made by the woman to terminate the soul that was to arrive and to beg its forgiveness. Women always feel relief after forgiveness. They carry their guilt for years and, after a certain amount of time, it transforms into an illness. Moreover, the unborn soul feels itself to be a rejected possibility during its first encounter with the physical world, and these feeling remains within them when they once again wish to enter a physical body. By breaking the connection, the mother receives forgiveness, and the new soul is freed from rejection and has the opportunity to enter into a physical body with another mother with love.

Sometimes abortions are unsuccessful, which likewise has an impact on the newborn child. Newborns in this case show resistance and anger towards their mother because they suffered from the fear that they would be rejected. Breaking this connection is necessary in order for the child to free itself of the unnatural fear of rejection and for the mother to forgive herself for the fact that she did everything she could to free herself from the child.

Given that people are subject to the influence of others, particularly people who did not receive enough love and understanding in childhood, they are drawn to groups and individuals who impress them with their powerful manner, and they believe these people when they say that they can, by changing their lifestyle, achieve positive changes. When they enter deeper into this, they discover that the opposite is true. This frequently happens to naive people who are not aware that, in addition to the positive, there are negative powers in the world and that their motives and beliefs cannot match their own. When a person like this realizes what has happened to them, they are usually already under the power of a group or an individual, and they do not have the strength to free themselves except with the help of another. It is necessary to understand that the collective energy of a group, or the powerful energy of an individual has an extremely strong effect on the energy body of the person who is drawn into it. For this reason, it is very difficult to release such a person from under this influence. This energy is always negative, given that groups and individuals feed on the energies of people with weaker energies and support their own egos and narcissism.

Some families carry a black cloud in their energy field, which is made up of the traumatic experiences experienced by groups or individuals who were once members of their family. These are usually caused by wars, earthquakes, and floods. Certain difficulties in the lives of members of such families prompt family memories of similar problems. Individuals can become so consumed by such old family traumas that they cannot face them. Such people are usually in a deep depression.

A child born into a particular family has genes that carry positive and negative family patterns. This is information about the traits and weaknesses that a child needs in order to learn in their new life. If a person consciously works on their negative traits and is aware of what they need to learn from them, they can speed this process up, and the negative traits can be reduced.

There is another thing that a person must free themselves from – we call it the inner enemy. It appears in dreams. The inner enemy is a combination of all those aspects of a particular person that constantly work against them and their wellbeing, however much they may struggle to improve. This figure takes on many forms: it can be male or female, young or old. Its appearance tells us that we are close to the root of the problem, most often the one that is the most important. The inner enemy usually brings along with it a large amount of negative energy, which is released after the inner enemy is defeated. Freeing oneself of this energy leads to a large amount of positive energy which appears in the form of understanding and acceptance, and the whole healing process is thus sped up.

The inner enemy is the cause of many nightmares in which it takes on the form of murderers, attackers, deceivers, doubters, ridiculers, or some other form that can prevent an individual from achieving their goal. These characters and forms are your hidden fears and dearly missed and un-comprehended feelings that return persistently with the honest desire to help you, for you to understand them, and to free yourself of them.

Aside from the inner enemy in human form, other negative forms can also appear which cause problems.

In dreams, such problems sometimes take on the form of an animal. The preferences of particular people for particular animals define them. The buffalo is known to represent stubbornness, pride, and conceit. The major characteristic of the sheep is stupidity, which prevents it from thinking logically and understanding. The cat is known for its cunning and its willingness to steal what it cannot have. The monkey is moody and inconstant, constantly leaping from one tree to another. The pig symbolizes avarice. The list is fairly long. Everyone should examine their unconscious before falling asleep so that their symbol may appear to them, and so that it can then be interpreted. These symbols are frequently expressed in a person's behavior. When one confronts them and accepts them, one overcomes them.

People can dream about their parents' houses after they separate from their parents or guardians. In dreams and lucid dreaming, this house frequently symbolizes the structure that the person has built around themselves in order to mark the territory or space that they take up in their own world, the space in which they live, move about, and exist.

Dreams can help us establish how we feel about ourselves and within ourselves and direct us towards the steps we have to take in order to uncover our true selves. It is first necessary to take a look at and understand oneself (to take a look in the mirror, as they say) in order to understand the behavior and actions of others.

People frequently dream about returning to their childhood home. This means that they are still unconsciously living in their old environment and that a part of them is still at the stage that they were at when they lived there.

Sometimes in dreams or lucid dreams a house will appear that seems attractive on the outside but is a huge mess on the inside. This is a shock for the person seeing such an image because it shows them their very selves, smiling on the outside but on the inside not everything is attractive. This shows the person how they present themselves to the world and that they must still resolve many things within.

Sometimes a person having a lucid dream will feel as though they are walking down a long, endless hallway. The hallway usually has numerous doors on either side. The hallway represents the path that the person takes when they wish to free themselves of habits, traumas, fears, rejection, unhappiness, loneliness, and other problems for which they do not know the cause and which make their path through life more difficult. The doors represent habits and other problems. The person frequently does not wish to open a single door because they fear change and because by changing their habits, they also change their lifestyle. When at last they make a decision, getting rid of habits one after the other, they free themselves of the shackles that bound them throughout their lives, and they begin to breathe freely and openly.

As soon as a child is born, it is exposed to a whole host of beliefs, expectations and models of behavior that define its future role as a man or woman in the social environment of the family. These patterns are transferred within the family from one generation to the next.

It is necessary to keep in mind the basic social values and adapt old-fashioned roles to the contemporary world. More and more, men and women do the same work together. Such a state of affairs can help both to develop their natural abilities, although the characteristics that are usually attributed to the opposite gender should not be forgotten in doing so. Both genders should achieve a balance between the head and the heart so that they can both think and feel equally well, which means balancing the masculine and feminine aspects within themselves.

One of the major causes of male chauvinism is the belief that cognitive and intellectual achievements are superior to all others. The consequence of this is the raising up of the intellect above man's other three functions: the senses, emotions, and intuition. However, all four functions are of equal importance and their individual development is essential for achieving completeness.

The chauvinistic approach of men in contrast to women, aside from favoring the intellect, includes the degradation of feeling. Men and women are not the same and they never will be, for good reasons, but both genders have masculine and feminine traits in various amounts and express them differently. Both genders should nurture the functions of the heart and feelings and should be able to express them. Both functions should cooperate in order for the person to achieve balance. They can thus establish their own truth and free themselves of narrow-minded views and superstitions that are rife in families and communities into which we were born and in which we live.

The majority of the patterns of thinking impressed upon us in childhood, primarily thanks to our parents and guardians are incorrect general ideas about other nations. Every nation is marked by patterns of behavior, action, culture, religion, and much besides. You have brought some of this with you into this life because during your previous incarnations you lived in various countries, societies, cultures, and religions. You have forgotten the larger part of this because, in being born on Earth, it is defined that a person does not remember their past lives and experiences. There are few people who are born on Earth and fated to recall a little of their past lives, and of course, there is a reason for this. The majority of people received all of their beliefs about other nations from parents and guardians.

Stereotypes about other nations are usually defined by characteristics such as miserliness, arrogance, flippancy, faltering, melancholia, conscientiousness, avarice, forcefulness, calculation, laziness, impulsiveness, and many others. If a person is born into these cultures that have a cultural stereotype attached to them, they will help that person to learn the lesson for which they were born precisely into that environment. Nobody has to identify with the negative stereotypes, just as everybody is free to break away from the negative aspects of their identity. Our identity is not determined by our belonging to a particular nation, just as our value, in the eyes of the world, is not determined by the amount of money we have, nor fame, beauty, or our level of refinement, but rather our positive attitude and positive behavior and a life lived in truth.

In order for a person to grow, to develop in a positive direction that they might in the end be in communion with and as one with God, God gives them countless possibilities, and one of these is reincarnation.

In every life, we borrow various things that we need for a limited time, as well as the people with whom we will have close relationships, positive and negative. By attaching ourselves to someone or something we create relationships with ourselves and with others. If people end the relationship with that which controls them and free themselves from further excessively restrictive attachments, they will be free at the moment of their death to leave behind their physical body and everything that tied them to that body throughout their lives. They can then experience a conscious death, discovering that they are alive since it is the soul that is eternal, and given that they have freed themselves of their physical bodies, they are also freed from its limitations. As the majority of people do not let go of their physical selves and things in their physical lives before they die, they are forced to return to a physical life in order to free themselves of this behavior and manner of thinking and to understand that they are in essence a soul that is reincarnated in a physical body. Frequent reincarnation allows them to get rid of all shackles, all cause and effect relationships on Earth.

A Technique for Ending Relationships and Connections with the Help of the All-Knowing and All-Pervasive Consciousness

When ending relationships with your former partner/s, it is essential to keep in mind that you must move everything from your immediate surroundings, your apartment, and your job that is connected to that individual because these things carry the energy of that person. This energy is, depending on the strength of your former relationship with your former partner, strong enough to destroy your relationship with your new partner.

When you begin using this technique, those people who know and can visualize will have strong visions. These visions can greatly frighten, surprise, and confuse you. Nothing negative can happen to you while using this technique, but it can direct you towards your attitude to someone and something and your attachment to someone or something.

People who were dependent on somebody or who were mistreated in any way could see themselves enveloped in large heavy chains and might imagine feeling as though everything is stifling them and that they can hardly breathe when using this technique. They will then realize that their relationship was in fact like this and that it is time to be free of it. There will be various other visions: that you are completely tied up with a rope with a ribbon on the top of your head or that you are connected via countless golden threads. All of these connections reflect your approach to that person or thing, and it is necessary to free yourself of them and relax and finally be free.

Those who do not have visions can imagine the whole process like in a dream or draw what they feel when practicing this technique on a piece of paper.

If you believe, because you have been told that you have some kind of genetic illness, that this means that the patterns of behavior have been handed down through the generations and have made their way to you as well, you can likewise free yourself from that using this technique, but it could frighten you greatly. Patterns of behavior that are transferred down the generations are exceptionally strong because they have been fed by many generations the attitudes of the surrounding environments and many others. You might see incredibly ugly creatures like something out of your worst nightmares. Do not give up; they cannot hurt you, and you can free yourself from this forever.

It is best to practice the technique for ending relationships not only with negative but with positive people and things as well because this shows that you are tied to somebody or something (for example, a pet) irrespective of the fact that such a relationship makes you feel happy and fulfilled. By breaking the connection, your relationship will become natural, which means that you will always be able to accept differences and changes without them prompting larger and longer traumas and frustrations.

The Technique

- Position yourself comfortably. Take a few deep breaths so that your physical body is as relaxed as possible and can come into closer contact with your higher self.
- Imagine a triangle (a geometric shape) with two corners resting on the ground and the top standing upright towards the sky.
- You are standing in one of the bottom corners, which is resting on the ground, and in the other is the person or thing with whom or with which you wish to break a connection.
- In the point that is facing the sky, place the being that is, for you, the most holy and positive and to which you usually turn for help from your religion. If you think this is not strong enough, none of the saints will hold it against you for this; simply ask God to help you and place Him at the top in your thoughts. (If you are drawing Him on paper, draw a white light, which is descending towards you and towards someone or something with whom/which you wish to break a connection.)
- Then study your connection: are you in chains, are you swimming in murky water, jumping around your axis? You can see all sorts of things

with your inner eye or with your senses if you are drawing.

- After that, watch the reaction of the person or thing that you placed in the triangle opposite you and with which you are breaking a connection. It can be both confusing and frightening because that person or thing will rebel on an energy level because it does not want change, given that it has been feeding off your energy the entire time. It may look like a beast with open jaws, a person dressed in black, an angry person; perhaps this kind of person will pull at strings or something else just to keep you at the same position in which it had been up till now. Do not be afraid but move on. This just shows you the unnaturalness and unhealthy attitude of your connection.
- This is when you should call on your saint or God Himself. They will appear as immeasurably powerful rays of positive energy. Alongside them you will begin to feel comfortable and relaxed in the certainty that they will take care of the business of breaking the connection instead of you in the most positive, natural and best manner for both sides. Wait and watch or sense what is happening. The side of the triangle opposite yours will change its attitude towards your intentions. It will first feel helpless, then confused, but it will eventually accept the change after all because it is positive and frees both sides from the bond and at the same time creates a healthy relationship between them.

- When the whole process is over, depending on your concentration and determination to resolve your problems, the end-result will be that there is no longer anything between you and that person or thing. In the triangle there will only be God, you, and that person separated.
- For those people who drew the breaking of the connection, take a pair of scissors and cut across the bottom line of the triangle that connected you and that other person or thing. Relax and try to sense how you feel now. You should begin to feel more and more relaxed.

Regression and Progression

This is a shallow hypnosis technique that is usually performed in pairs, which means you and a person that you trust. You then lie down on a flat surface, a bed for instance, and the trusted person leads you through the whole process. The trusted person can be your best friend or a hypnotherapist. Your friend is a person who has a similar energy to yours, so it is quite likely that you have more faith in them than you do in a stranger.

The process itself consists of totally relaxing the body from the top of the head to the tips of the toes, so that your physical body is completely relaxed, and you are in a state halfway between sleeping and waking. At this time your consciousness is completely open, and you are completely aware of your surroundings. Given that your physical body is in this state, you are slightly stiff but you quickly adapt to this state, given that you can move unhindered; it is only necessary that these movements are very gentle and slow so that your physical body can remain in a light trance.

Your friend or the hypnotherapist asks questions in order to uncover the cause of your current illnesses and frustrations, and you, in this light trance, see images or even a film showing what caused this situation and the reasons for this. You do not need to recount this to anyone but keep it for yourself. You participate in the whole process verbally irrespective of the fact that you cannot ask yourself questions because of the state of your consciousness but rather those questions must be asked by your friend or the hypnotherapist. If something interests you, feel free to indicate to your friend or hypnotherapist which question you would like answered, and they will ask it and you will receive an answer.

If you are not immediately able to see the images, do not lose hope; this is just a small, beginner's failure. If your head begins to hurt because of the tension and the anticipation, you can gently end the whole process by moving your toe, or you can ask your friend or hypnotherapist to end the whole process.

After the whole process finishes stretch gently and relax so that your body can once again adapt to the present. This adaptation can last up to twenty minutes, and during this time, replay the images and films in your head so that you can later write them down and link them with the situations in which you find yourself.

Give yourself time to adjust.

Just one more small but incredibly important note: everything that you do must be for your own well-being and in your absolute best interests. It must express love towards you yourself or you will not receive that which you are searching for, and you will become more frustrated than you were before – not because of the process of hypnosis but because of your unrealistic and negative expectations.

Regression

Regression means returning to past lives in order to uncover connections with things, people, events, and your interest in particular things that define you in this life.

- People are born with a particular energy pattern, which carries within itself a part of the feelings, responsibilities and interests which were experienced and lived in one or perhaps more than one past life. It frequently happens that a person feels a drive to do charity work exclusively with animals, which can be tied to the fact that they lived in a tribe and from hunting and that they felt an immeasurable respect for and valued the animals that gave their lives in order for that person to live. In addition, you can see that you were somewhere in some country an alchemist, which is why you are interested in science in this life.

- The next thing that you can discover is the reason why you received precisely the kind of character that you have. If you were a cruel leader in a past life, you will probably be a follower who is mistreated and oppressed by his leader, so that the cause and effect relationship may come full circle. Or if you were a Crusader in one of your past lives, you will probably have had enough of blood for your next few lifetimes, and in this life you will choose the role of a doctor in order to clear away the consequences of something that was probably imposed upon you at that time but at the same time you also believed in those ideals at that time.

- There is also a link with the illnesses that you encounter in this life, which are always tied to some kind of unresolved events and situations. Constant, strong migraines can be connected to an affair in one of your past lives, irrespective of the positive attitudes towards the person in that life. The very understanding that this is wrong and the very attitude of the society of the time can create problems for you that you need to resolve in this life. This part deals with feelings that you brought with you from your past lives. By resolving various kinds of feelings in this life, you free yourself from illness and the health-related problems that you brought with you in your energy field.

- The final thing is your connection with the people that you meet in this life. You have already met in various roles in at least one of your former lives all of the people you will meet in this life. This happens so that you can experience various relationships and accept the differences. Such relationships are mother/daughter, father/son, grandmother/grandson, and all other possible combinations within the family.

- The second form is that of a partnership. Usually, partners merely swap genders but always remain together except that various situations occur to them in order for them to grow and understand one another. You can have a partner now with whom you got on very well in several lives and your relationship is harmonious in this life, but you can also get a partner with whom you had particular conflicts and with whom you now live in order to understand one another, overcome all differences, and consequently understand why you are together. Resolving all your differences leads to release, forgiveness, and freedom, and those souls then no longer come together and do not enter into the karmic cycle of rebirth.

Progression

Progression is seeing future events from the current position of your behavior and way of thinking. There is no space or time here, and you can therefore see yourself, perhaps with more lines on your face or a different posture, in order to determine the possibility of the period when, given the current moment, this particular event might occur in the future.

The possibility exists that you might see, if it interests you, your next life, although this is rare given that individuals' ways of thinking are very changeable and in fact change from moment to moment.

- The extent to which your current path via your thoughts is defined will be your future on the personal and professional level. If you are thinking about changing your job and are in fact not considering the same profession, it can happen that, if it is more energetically powerful in your thoughts (which means you are already transforming that profession into something material, even if you are not aware of this) that you see yourself ending up in a completely different job and that you will be fulfilled by it. A sudden love can also appear because you have already formed it in your thoughts by describing the person, their character, their appearance, and everything that is important to you.

- Just as your way of thinking is defined in the present so are the possibilities of you falling ill and the problems that these kinds of thoughts project. If you have not formed a good relationship with your children, in the future they might ignore you and you would suffer because of this. Alternatively, your constant announcements that everything is on you and that you cannot trust anyone to take over anything because you have trained that other person to become used to you doing everything can in the future lead to high blood pressure because of the pressure that you have, over the past few decades, placed upon yourself. You might see this as images of yourself constantly visiting the doctor, measuring your blood pressure, and taking medications.

- Given that you can change everything, progression is an answer to your current thinking, and you receive these kinds of pictures. You can also see potential traumatic future events that are related to you and which you can change if you change your way of thinking after progression. Just by doing so, the next time you enter into progression, that event will no longer exist, or it will be completely softened. Everything depends on you. You create your destiny in this moment. Decide what kind you would like and follow that path.

- A person who has a great many problems, suffering, sorrow, and other situations that make their life harder (everyone is given only as much as they can handle!) in this life can see why so much of this has built up, understand the purpose of these events and situations in this life, and, by resolving everything, and understand who they in fact are. Nobody is punishing you with any kind of problems; rather, they are given to you because you are in such an environment and in such a place that you will be able to reach the answers that will help you solve them. The more sufferings you have in life and the more of these you understand and resolve, the more you release yourself from a certain number of the lives that you were given in the cause and effect relationship wheel because you were reincarnated on Earth.

Part II
What You Are Given at Birth

Astral Projection – Projection into a Subtle Dimension

Astral projection is the projection of one part of an energy body. This part is that energy part of your material body that is wrapped around your mental, psychic, and physical bodies. It is the energy part of your body that enters the astral plane. People have a fear of death and so think if their soul is out of their body, they will die; they think that their soul leaves them. In this case it does not happen. The body dwells in the energy part of the body that is related to your two higher bodies: the spiritual body and the soul. That part is given to you at birth and does not leave you until you decide to leave your physical body. This means that when you enter into an astral projection you are not dead, nor can you be. Your material body continues to perform its function. You are not exposed to any undesirable situations because your material body is safe, and whenever it is necessary, it calls on the energy body that is in the projection, is back in your material body in moments, and is joined with the energy body that is related to the soul and the spirit. They once more form a whole.

For babies this is a normal state, given that upon entering into an astral projection they feel a freedom from the limits of their physical body. They do this almost every time they sleep. It has been known to happen, albeit rarely, that this part of the energy no longer wishes to return to the material body for reasons known only to the soul and so takes with it that part of the energy that is related to the soul and the spirit. When this happens, the baby experiences physical death. Such phenomena happen up until the baby's first year of life, after which they no longer occur.

In childhood, above the age of three years, this is still a very frequent occurrence. Children relax in this way and feel carefree, even though their parents and guardians are already trying to place them into family and social molds. Later, this part is lost because of the weight of the molds into which they are placed.

In the very act of freeing yourself from the mold, you also free your soul and it once again begins to revel in that for which it entered a physical body to begin with. This is when the possibility of once again consciously entering the astral plane returns to you.

In the process of splitting energies for the purposes of astral projection, a division of consciousness occurs but only fictitiously. This means that one part of the consciousness, which is presented as a whole, remains in the material body (relating to the spirit and soul), and the other part of the consciousness goes with the other part of the energy (relating to the material body), which is also a whole. These two wholes are linked by a so-called silver cord, a thin energy line. In this way, everything that you experience on the astral plane is collected as experience and knowledge in your material body.

On the astral plane, there are no feelings, and it is absolutely clear to you that everything you see and experience is connected to you, but you do not feel real emotions, sorrows, joys or any others, only fictitious feelings. In addition, you can also meet other beings during your time on the astral plane. You communicate with them telepathically and therefore understand one another perfectly.

People who are not prepared – which means that they do not believe in it or are scared – are not permitted to remember that they experienced something like this, so that they might be protected from their fear. The more responsive a person is to accepting themselves and everything that has been given to them in this material body, the more open they are, and they have a greater chance of remembering that they were on the astral plane, what they experienced, and how they liked it.

Children who enter the astral plane are completely protected from the strange beings that might appear on the astral plane.

Beginners who wish to once again consciously enter the astral plane as adults begin with a certain fear, and when they are successful, so-called lower vibrational beings, who are only visible to humans on the astral plane, can create panicked fear without reason. Given that they are from the second dimension (humans are in the third) their only amusement is frightening those who are insecure because they feed off such energy. The energy of people who meet these kinds of beings finds itself, in an instant, in its material body, full of terror with a beating heart and other symptoms. It is easy to get rid of such beings; the beginner only has to be aware of their weakness and it is enough to simply send them a positive thought telepathically because beings from the lower, or second dimension (2D) are afraid of this. The beginner can also keep following his or her path without paying these beings any attention.

For the clarification cause the explanation of dimensions. The first dimension (1D) is the lowest dimension. This dimension is the energy of thought, the first energy, which is the spark of the beginning of creation. The second dimension (2D) is the energy of creating the first material things. We and all what is on the Earth are in the third dimension (3D). In the third dimension starts the opportunity to grow souls. The highest dimension is known as the ninth dimension (9D). There are highly intelligent beings who are pure love energy and who are the nearest to God. All beings created by God need to pass the whole transformation.

Those who are not strangers to this will never meet beings from the lower dimensions, only from their own or higher.

There are two kinds of experiences on the astral plane. One is the zone of the current situation and the second is true astral projection.

The zone of the current situation is a zone within the Earth's atmosphere and is therefore subject to space and time. You can remain on the astral plane within this zone for twenty minutes at most and still remember everything that you experienced outside your material body afterwards. Here you can meet the energies of your friends, business partners, and others, and nobody will be aware of this because as I have already mentioned, people enter the astral plane unconsciously and remain there unconsciously. You can visit countries or read books in languages that are foreign to you because you read them telepathically (which means that you understand everything). You can visit someone who is very close to you and have excellent relations with that person, although they are far away, and you are not able to visit them physically.

During a projection, you may look at your energy hands, and they may disappear from the fingers towards the palm; when this happens, look away, then back again, and your energy hands will return and then disappear after some time. This is a normal and natural phenomenon.

True astral projection is a projection outside the Earth's atmosphere. Time does not exist there, so you can spend a considerable amount of time there – or until your alarm clock rings and you are returned in an instant to your material body. In this way, you can very easily explore the Universe. For projections where your body is energetically powerful, your energy shape on the astral plane is not lost, but it can change according to your mental wishes.

When entering the astral plane, you take on the form that you created in your mind, so you defined yourself that way. This does not have to be the shape of your physical body.

Given that everything is achieved through practice, particularly when someone has already established certain beliefs in you, you first have to understand that these beliefs are unacceptable and inappropriate. For most people, projection occurs while they are in an alpha state, i.e. the time between sleeping and waking before morning, usually between four and six o'clock. The body is then rested and relaxed. This means that the body is sleeping lightly and usually only projects its energy outside the material body.

Projection is also possible when a person is completely awake. For some people it is natural and is therefore easier for them to achieve, while the majority of people will have to put in a great deal of hard work.

You will know whether you have ever been on the astral plane, which the majority of people believe to be impossible if you are not dead, when you recall if you have ever felt as though you were falling in your sleep, or if you have ever dreamed that you are flying. These are the most common phenomena.

On the astral plane, your energy body is free from all limitations, so you can pass through solid physical objects. You can pass through the Earth, or you can go to whichever corner of the Universe you like best. Your energy cord, which links your energy body on the astral plane with your physical body and which is lying peacefully in bed or wherever else, is limitless.

The Technique for Entering the Astral Plane from an Alpha State

The easiest method, which will not always be successful, is to say a prayer before falling asleep that you remember everything that happens to you while you are asleep. If you wish to work on getting to know this part of you, this is a method by which, through practice, you can enter the astral plane in a light sleep (alpha state) and later remember everything that you experienced.

Be disciplined. Eat very little in the evening, just enough to satisfy your hunger if you feel any.

Go to bed, if it is at all possible, at the same time every day, and wake up at about the same time every morning.

Keep a notebook and pencil close to your bed.

- Every evening pray to God that you will remember everything that you will dream or experience while your material body is asleep.
- If you awake during the night, remain still for a moment and try to recall what you dreamt or what happened to you just before you woke up. Write everything down, both dreams and possible projections, because this can sometimes be mixed up into one experience.
- Write down your dreams every morning, which means that you wake up every morning determined to know what you dreamed and experienced.
- During the day try to occasionally think about your material body and relax it. Simply sit up straight on your chair or stand or walk. Then focus on your breathing and the way you breathe; concentrate on your breathing and think only about your breathing. This will help you stop your thoughts from wandering.
- Throughout the day, ask yourself a few times if this is a dream. Am I dreaming this? Given that you frequently relive the events from the previous day in your dreams, this is an exercise for concentration.
- Eat light meals throughout the day until you are satisfied of course. Do not consume un-

necessarily heavy food (meat and fish), not in large quantities at least.
- Before sleeping do breathing exercises (meditation) in order to unburden yourself of the energies of the events that you experienced that day.

Sooner or later, you will be successful. The stronger your faith, the sooner the possibility of experiencing astral projection from a light sleep will open before you.

Through practice, prayer, and focus, you will be able to reach the point where, when you find yourself on the astral plane, you yourself can decide what you want to see, visit or learn.

The Technique for Entering the Astral Plane While Your Material Body Is Awake

For some people this is natural, so that they can, from any place at all, create a situation in which their material body's energy can be projected onto the astral plane. Those for whom this is not natural have to put in a little hard work if they wish to enter the astral plane while they are conscious.

In order to make the projection easier for yourself, you need to increase the amount of energy in the body. The exercise for increasing your energy is such that you go from every part of your body and focus your thoughts on that region. You begin with the big toe of one foot, and then move on to the next toe, and so on in order; then onto the foot, heel, calf, knee, and everything in order past the organs and the skin until you come to the scalp. In order to make the flow of energy to particular parts of the body easier when the power of your thoughts is not yet powerful enough, lightly touch those places with your index finger or make circular motions. Men should motion in a clockwise direction and women in the opposite, counterclockwise direction, when on the right side of the body; on the left side the opposite applies.

When you have mastered this technique, you will begin to feel warmth in the part that you have touched with your hand or thoughts. After this, you learn to direct energy through the body. In this way, you can also achieve a stronger energy activity in the body, which takes care of energy blockages in the body. Energy blockages are places in which illness on the lowest, physical level manifests. You first lead the energy through the first five energy regions. These are the regions of the first five energy centers. When you stabilize the energy, which means that you feel gentle, comfortable warmth in your entire body except in the head, you can begin leading energy into the head.

Do not try to achieve the energy that you do not have in a very short time frame, which means long-term, daily practice in order not to do your body more harm than good. The harm that you can do to yourself is mental and emotional destabilization.

Practice every day for no more than twenty minutes. When you sense, after a few weeks, that your energy is stabilizing, begin practicing daily for no more than thirty minutes. Practice daily, and even when you have mastered the technique it should last no longer than sixty minutes (one hour).

Always, absolutely always, ask for help and guidance from your higher consciousness, God, because then you will always achieve what you need to and what is best for you. Approach this very seriously.

Everything that you do seriously, conscientiously, and under the guidance of your higher consciousness will help you to free yourself from negative energy and bring your physical body into balance.

After doing the technique for increasing the energy of the body, relax, and do breathing exercises for at least twenty minutes in the beginning. Later you will not need this because your consciousness will automatically react to your thoughts, and your physical body will relax in an instant).

Place a notebook and pencil beside you.

- Relax completely in your armchair, so that the angle of the armchair is under about 140 degrees. (It is harder to fall asleep in an armchair than it is in a bed). Be careful to stabilize your head, so that it will not fall while you are completely relaxed.
- Sense your energy body.
- Feel how the energy of your body is increasing more and more.

- Feel the energy of your material body separating from the energy body of your soul and spirit.
- Feel how your consciousness is separating into two equal halves and at the same time forms a whole.
- One part of your energy is slowly separating from the other. Here you might experience a powerful beating in your chest, which you should immediately ignore because it is not real. You might hear an unbearable noise, which is not tied to the physical world. You can ignore this too. Irrespective of the phenomena in your body or if you hear any kind of noise outside your body, these are not real phenomena but your imagination, which is trying to tell you that you are not ready yet. Irrespective of everything, try to stay calm and relaxed. This part of the problem will pass. You can also call on your higher consciousness to help you.
- Techniques for separating the energy of the material body from the energy of the soul and mind can be tug-of-war (when with your imaginary hands you climb a rope out of your physical body towards the ceiling) or climbing a ladder (when with your imaginary hands and legs you climb a ladder towards the ceiling). These are the two techniques that are the most popular and that have yielded the best results.
- You are outside of your physical body.

You then choose where you will go and what you will do using your thoughts, all in a period of twenty minutes, in order to return consciously with a new experience.

This is a natural way in which the soul is freed from the energies of the material body that weigh it down because in this way the energy of the material body is cleansed by the energy that it receives from the absolute consciousness (from whence it came when it entered a physical body). This is a natural and all-but-everyday process, particularly for people who have withdrawn so much into their own ego that they do not see anyone or anything except themselves.

On the astral plane, you understand that the center of your existence is the soul and not your physical body, and this knowledge itself leads you to stop fearing physical death.

Reiki

Reiki is energy of light and love, a healing energy that is woven into the energy of your body. Nobody has to give it to you through an initiation because you already have it, but in order to begin using it, you must know that it exists. Simply by knowing that it exists, it is necessary to know how to use it properly. This is an extremely strong energy for which a person must be prepared, meaning that they are on the path towards cleansing their physical body in order to lift up the soul. Until the person is ready, they do not even have the ability to use it. It is energy of your higher consciousness to which you must demonstrate, through your relationship with yourself, and show that you are prepared for it.

Reiki is an absolutely positive, intelligent energy, which in and of itself does not allow you to do any kind of harm to yourself.

Given that it is completely tied to the absolute consciousness, reiki is a healing energy at the deepest level. This means that it heals all your traumas from your past life, your mental and psychic body (illness on the physical level is a reflection of an energy attitude on the mental and psychical level), and it can therefore heal a person absolutely without any unwanted repercussions and without the possibility of the illness ever returning. The condition is that the person being healed listens and obeys the master or teacher in terms of how they have to change their behavior towards themselves and others in order to stay in this kind of new healthy state.

After a healing done by a true master, a teacher of reiki who cleanses your body using energy directly from the cells of your body, a turbulent reaction takes place in your body. This reaction is caused by the fact that the body protests and is confused by the sudden, powerful change. Such a bodily reaction lasts a very short time, and after a short period the body happily adapts to the new situation, works with you, and helps you on your path to healing your body on all three levels: mental, psychic and physical. The reactions usually appear after a few days. You can develop a temperature of forty degrees Celsius/one hundred and four Fahrenheit, which cannot, of course, be decreased by any kind of medicine because it is not of a physical nature. When you have this kind of temperature, you feel well except for the fact that you feel sleepier than usual. This kind of temperature usually lasts a day or two at most. You can have diarrhea that lasts up to five days and strong sweats that usually smell very bad. (Sweat on its own does not smell. Sweat smells only as a warning that there is some kind of problem and illness in the physical body.) You can have angry outbursts or burst into tears because the organism is cleansing itself. This is good for you, of course, but warns those around you because it could be very confusing for them. The angry outbursts are not directed at anybody, which means nobody found in your vicinity, but are a feeling that you are expelling from yourself by screaming, which is not directed at anybody.

Many people wish to be initiated, that is to reach a certain level of reiki for a particular sum of money. Given that we live in a material world, people who are dubbed masters and teachers of reiki will happily do this because for many this is their only source of income. In order to reach the master and teacher level, a person has to pass through various cleansings and be completely open to their self. There are very few people like this. You will be able to sense immediately people who are on the right path towards this knowledge. Just trust your intuition. Such people can help you. The people to whom you can turn are people who are primarily mentally, psychically, and physically healthy, who live in healthy surroundings and who create healthy surroundings wherever they are. People who wish to make improvements on their life's journey seek them out in their vicinity. Such people will help you for free, but they will never allow you to become attached to them. Attachment means attachment to the physical, and those who have already gone through this will never return to their old state but will move forward towards self-fulfillment.

Money has a low energy value and a true master knows this and never accepts it to avoid doing himself harm. He will help you from the heart and with a great deal of love, which will be useful for both him and you. It will be useful for him inasmuch as he will be fulfilled beyond measure by his love towards you and himself and useful to you because you will discover the truth about a problem, understand it, and resolve it. The cycle of this illness or problem will thus be ended and it will no longer appear. In doing this you raise your energy, cleanse your energy field, and become a healthy person, a person who has ever more understanding towards themselves and others, and as this kind of person, you begin to accept and love yourself.

Through the very act of initiation, the person uncovers symbols in their body, which are immeasurably filled with positive energy. If the individual does not behave in keeping with the words of the master, the teacher – which means the individual has to work on cleansing the body, ceasing to swear, ceasing to eat meat and fish, practicing healthy sex, ceasing to drink alcohol, ceasing to smoke, and all other unhealthy habits – the body cannot be cleansed because you do not allow it to. Your reiki therefore closes and waits for another opportunity. Everyone thinks that through initiation they will receive and retain their reiki and that they will be able to use it whenever they feel like it. They say that there is a time for everything, and the same applies in this case.

It can happen that nothing positive occurs in their physical body. Their problems and illnesses are not healed, and they are angry that they paid money and that clearly, so they think, they did not receive an adequate service in return. But initiation gives you only the possibility of healing, and it is up to you whether you will accept this gladly and head down the path of truth and personal change or if everything will remain the same. When your master or teacher initiates you, they always tell you that you have to work on yourself for at least twenty-one days, which is of course short time, but in this way, they wish to force you to be disciplined and to discipline your body and your way of life.

Symbols make your intention to cleanse yourself easier. If you accept the fact that you have to give up only that which you already know is doing you harm, this means that you are heading down the path towards developing the truth about yourself and your selfhood. This is when those symbols will be of immeasurable aid because you show them your faith in your welfare and your love towards yourself.

If the master, the teacher, does not develop themselves within reiki, then they will remain on the first level of healing, that is, the laying of hands on the body of the person they are healing. In these cases, give that kind of master or teacher a wide berth because they could not even help themselves and will therefore not be able to help you either.

A true master, a true teacher, will know your full diagnosis from the point of view of energy with one examination of your body, which means that they will know in which parts of your body the blockages that have led to particular problems or diseases are located. They do not need diagnoses from doctors of Western medicine.

In addition, a true master, a true teacher, heals from a distance because they know that everything is energy and that nothing is outside of energy. In this case, he condenses energy on the energy plane and sends it along with immeasurable love to the person who requires it. Given that energy is the consciousness out of which everything is created, the person is healed.

The master or teacher is not permitted to heal every person, and they know this and will politely decline your request. The reason for this is that they know whether the person is prepared for a change within themselves or not. If they are not prepared, they must be given time to develop the desire for change, and the master or teacher is then allowed to offer them help.

If the person who needs help cannot ask for it themselves, because they are in a coma or in an unconscious or similar state, the master or teacher can ask their soul if it wants help. The soul, which knows what is best for the physical body, will reply in keeping with this.

Since reiki is given to us at birth, it is useful for pregnant women and small children and for every age group. You also do not need a master or a teacher to initiate you. This is yet another reason why a true master, a true teacher, will not ask for payment for their services.

The five symbols of reiki used for treating the body are known exactly; it is known how they work on what part of the energy body and that you can always use them when you are ready.

Ask God to guide you as to whether you are ready to receive the symbols; if you are you will feel gentle warmth on your palm or both palms. When you receive the symbols yourself or when you receive them from your master, your teacher, then it is essential that you search for guidance from your higher self. It knows best whether you are prepared to move forward and by how much. Do not hurry, give yourself time, and everything will work in your favor.

Many initiated people, and those that are convinced they have set out on a spiritual path, ignore their physical body; they ignore its mental, psychic, and physical needs. They begin reading books that are for the most part not appropriate for the developmental stage they are currently at because they read everything they are given. The majority of books that deal with spirituality, for the most part, do not explain the harmful effects of people focusing only on the one spiritual aspect of themselves while the other aspects that together form the body and which all need to be balanced between themselves, are ignored. Everything you read you must read with an open heart. For everything you read, you need to ask your higher self if it is good for you and if everything that is offered in the material you read is the truth. I recommend that you carefully and precisely develop and read only self-help books that explain to you your approaches and your reactions to particular external stimuli, whether it deals with feelings or events. Simply by opening up towards your higher self, the right opportunities and the right books for you will appear, the right people will enter into your life. The right situations that you will be able to understand, the right positive relations between people that you have not yet felt (or not felt to that great an extent), the right people who will offer you care, love, empathy, and help when you need it and in the manner that is best for you will come. Believe.

For people who have set out on a so-called spiritual path, because they do not think about their physical body, they have a problem – a big problem where the energy of their body, is not properly distributed throughout the entire body and begins to climb into the upper energy centers, which means into the head. This leads to disharmony in the body. The individual feels as though they are floating, and they are not aware of real-life situations. This leads to a slight mental disorder. Such an individual can only be helped by lowering their energy to distribute it properly throughout the body.

Anybody who is close to them and who wishes to help that person out of love can do this for them. The method involves placing one palm on the tailbone (the lower part of the spine) of that person and the other on the top of the cervical spine. Ask God to harmonize the energy and He will do so. Do this every day, up to three times a day, until you feel soft warmth in both palms. Then ask the person you were helping if they feel that warmth through their whole spine. If they reply in the affirmative, the process is complete. It is a warning not to do this to yourself anymore.

The first symbol is *Cho-ku-rei,* which in translation means "God is here". This symbol purifies your physical body. Initiation into this symbol teaches you how to lay hands on the body. The laying on of hands is done on that part of the body for which you know there is an energy blockage. It eases and harmonizes the flow of energy through the body.

The second symbol is *Sei-he-kei* which in translation means "God and man become one." This symbol purifies your psychic body, which means that, with this new symbol, one goes a step further. By laying hands, you cleanse and balance the energies that relate to your physical and psychic body and harmonize them into one whole, one energy body.

The third symbol is *Hon-sha-ze-sho-nen* which in translation means "The God in me reaches out to the God in you to bring us to enlightenment and peace."

This symbol purifies your mental body. By laying on hands you balance all three energy fields that relate to your material body, your mental, psychic, and physical into one harmonious whole, one energy body.

The fourth symbol is *Dai-ko-myo* which in translation means "the temple of the great shining light in which man's consciousness and God become one." This symbol links the energy of your material body with the energy of your soul into one harmonious whole, one energy body.

The fifth symbol is *Raku*, which in translation means "completion/fulfillment, reaching nirvana (total bliss, unity with God)." This symbol links the energy of your spirit with the energy of your soul and your material body into one indivisible, perfect, absolute whole, one energy body.

Use what you have been given by God and follow Him.

Clairvoyance

Clairvoyance is correctly foreseeing future events. This largely refers to individuals themselves, who are mostly clairvoyant in terms of their own selves, and then their closest family members. People who deeply believe in their intuition and who accept and know themselves very well use their power of clairvoyance more than others do.

The gland in the body (head) that makes clairvoyance possible is the pineal gland, the so-called third eye, or inner eye.

Clairvoyance is energy. Given that it is energy, you can shape it.

You frequently say to yourself that something will happen for some reason or other, which either happens in the way that you imagined or in a similar way. Later a person tells themselves, "I knew that would happen. I had a premonition."

Psychics are people who look at your energy field when you come to them to determine a particular problem or disease in your physical body. Every psychic sees this field differently: some see it in colors, some in clouds, and some in black-and-white. Some psychics will see images or films in your energy field, while some will close their eyes and see your problems with their third eye.

Every psychic sees the situation from the present, current state of your energy field. If the development of your personality will continue to head in the same direction – which is all but impossible because you experience various situations every day that force a change in your way of thinking and thus your energy field as well – what the psychic tells you will most probably be the truth in the present moment but not for your future. The very act of changing yourself, even in the minimal field, leads to your energy field changing around you and your future along with it.

This means that if a psychic has told you that you will, as it currently stands, likely develop an illness or experience an accident in the future, you can, through positive changes to your attitude and behavior, make a positive change in your energy field and to events in your future as well. You change your fate. Everything is down to you.

For those who look to a psychic to help them with a current illness, the psychic can see the event that triggered the development of that illness. By cleansing yourself, through understanding the situation and forgiveness, you purify your energy field and thus treat and heal the illness that you have.

Whenever you ask a psychic about something, always focus on yourself alone. Do not include in the so-called "seeing process" your partners, family, or work colleagues because you are the important one. By changing yourself, you change the situation around you.

There are two very simple techniques for improving and strengthening your psychic powers.

The first technique is looking at a flower through your inner eye.

- First decide what kind of flower you would like to see with your third eye. This should be a flower you like. The easiest way is to first draw that flower on a piece of paper or to have it close by. Try to think of as simple a flower as possible, so that it is easier for you to concentrate and visualize.

- Relax and inhale and exhale a few times in order to relax your body and to connect with your higher consciousness. Settle yourself comfortably in a chair or armchair. To begin with, physically look at the flower you drew or have it nearby.
- Slowly close your eyes and try to imagine and see it with your inner eye.
- Look at its petals, stem, and leaves.
- Assume that every petal on your flower represents one area that interests you, your job, your partner, money, luck, and everything that interests you. There are as many petals on the flower as you wish there to be. In the same way decide what the stem, leaves, even the thorns (if you have imagined them on your flower) represent for you.
- On a piece of paper, write down which petal will represent a particular idea, person or body part – whatever truly interests you.
- With your eyes closed, first examine the entire flower together with the stem and leaves. It represents you yourself. How you are feeling in this particular moment physically, psychically, and mentally. Look at the flower to see if it has gained or lost color, if the stem has changed from healthy green to brown and dry, or if it has even decayed. Look at the leaves to see if they

have some color or if here, too, there has been a change.

- Write everything down. It will be easier to explain everything to yourself later. If you are alone while doing this exercise, constantly opening your eyes and making notes will not decrease your concentration, and you can therefore continue with the exercise unimpeded.
- On a piece of paper, note the size, shape, strength, weakness, and all other changes in the flower's petals. You might not be able to find it because you have either destroyed that part of yourself, or you have repressed to such an extent that you are afraid for it to return to the surface once more, or it simply isn't there yet.
- When you are done with the exercise, ask God to help you disentangle, resolve, help you get healthy, help you make a dream job a reality, or help you make an as-yet imaginary creative solution a reality. Feel yourself placing the flower in God's hands and how everything is resolved in the way that is best for you.

The second technique is watching a television screen with your inner eye.

- Relax and inhale and exhale a few times in order to relax your body and to connect with your higher consciousness and concentrate better.
- Look at the television screen for some time or draw it on a piece of paper.
- Concentrate, relax, and then slowly close your eyes.

- Look at the television screen with your inner eye.
- Allow your consciousness to show you a particular image on the screen. If a symbol appears, which may be in the form of a flower, animal, letters, or sign, ask your higher consciousness to explain it to you.
- In this way you receive an answer to a question you did not ask but which is at this moment very important for your present and future life.
- At the end, you must thank God for the advice offered and for directing you towards the right path.

You can also do this technique with the help of the questions that interest you. You may receive answers that are, at your current level of development and in relation to your current way of thinking, completely unacceptable to you. If they have been shown to you, know that they are truthful. Ask for them to explain themselves to you. If they do not explain themselves this means that you are not yet ready for the answer; if they explain themselves, you know what you need to do.

You might see persons and recognize them, but they look extremely well and happy, or the complete opposite. Ask your higher consciousness what the reason for this is, and you will receive the answer in the form of an image, images, or film.

Telepathy

The word "telepathy" comes from two separate Greek words where *tele* means "at a distance" and *pathy* means "to feel". Telepathy means sensing someone or something at a distance, that is, communication at a distance without using verbal speech.

The pineal gland, the third eye, is the center you use to communicate at a distance.

Telepathy is the sending of energy to a distant point. Individuals communicating with each other need to be on more or less the same frequency in order to receive the signals that they send to one another.

Up until their third year of life, children communicate telepathically amongst themselves, later this way of communicating is lost given that they begin using speech.

It is said that mothers understand their babies even though they do not communicate using speech.

People who have been married a long time already know what the other is thinking and what they are going to do.

People who are deeply in love know what suits their partners without them having to say it.

Some people warn their nearest and dearest about dangers using their thoughts because they intuitively sense the danger and therefore send their loved ones messages from a distance.

Sometimes a person whom you have not spoken to for a long time and about whom you have been thinking about intensively recently calls you.

Some people can on occasion read the thoughts of the person with whom they are speaking.

There are countless examples and situations you come across every day, and you are not aware of them.

Telepathy can be sensory, vocal, or visual.

Sensory telepathy is when you sense another person from a distance. Often this is their warmth under normal circumstances, but you can feel spasms in certain parts of the body, shivers that you know do not come from yourself alone. This is when you know that something has happened to that other person and that by sending them the energy of love you can always help them.

Verbal telepathy is when a person hears voices in their head which appear like verbal conversations between people.

Visual telepathy is when you see certain images or films in your inner eye, and they are only connected to the person with whom you are in telepathic contact.

A training technique:

- Find a person to whom you are close and with whom you have long been in a harmonious relationship. This can be a friend, partner, or someone who understands you and you them.
- Select a peaceful place where nobody will disturb you for at least thirty minutes.
- Do some relaxation exercises.
- Sit on chairs or armchairs so that you are comfortable, one across from the other.
- Relax.
- Agree that you will think about a particular thing, for instance a pencil.
- One person should think about the length, shape, or color – whatever crosses their mind in relation to a pencil – and project it (send it to the other person). Before projecting it, the object must be completely and firmly defined in the head of that person.
- The second person should try and sense and see in their inner eye exactly how the imaginary pencil sent by the other person looks.

Sleep and Dreams

Sleep is a rest for your physical body, but it is not so for either your psychic, mental, emotional, or spiritual bodies. All the other bodies are extremely active at this time. This is why dreams appear. People who have had an intense day and very little sleep usually do not remember them because then their physical body needs a stronger rest in a short period and so it relaxes more deeply. People who have a disciplined sleeping rhythm usually remember their dreams in the early morning, between four and six o'clock when the body is very relaxed and the consciousness very strong. At this time, it is useful to write down these dreams because they always have some kind of message. Immediately after waking up, stay in bed for a few minutes and think about all the dreams that you remember. As soon as you get up, write down your dreams because you will forget them just ten minutes later. The reason is that in those first ten waking minutes, your unconscious is still strong. After that there is a change into a conscious state.

Dreams frequently help to make situations in which you find yourself clearer or explain the emotions that you feel. With all dreams, it is necessary to take control of them. You need to become aware that they are only dreams that want to show you something and in doing so help you.

It is necessary to understand that the dream is your reality when your physical body is resting. Through your dreams, you experience all emotions, events, and situations unconsciously.

When you dream only pleasant dreams, you will know that you have gotten rid of all your fictional enemies, including people, frustrations, problems, diseases, and unwanted emotions.

There are four kinds of dreams.

Nightmares are a mixture of imagination, situations you have found yourself in, terrifying beings that represent your emotions, frustrations, or problems. They usually chase you, and you run away and wake up in a cold sweat or with a beating heart. Try to take control over your dreams. Turn around and you will see who or what is chasing you. If it has a face that you can see, it may be familiar or unfamiliar. A familiar face is related to a person that you know and with whom you may not even have been aware that you have a mutual problem. An unfamiliar face might be one of your hidden negative feelings or frustrations. Try to get a look at the facial expression. Perhaps it will reveal to you what it represents. Look at the whole situation and event and then write it down after you wake up. Later, when you are awake, ask your higher consciousness to explain to you what that person from your dreams represents.

Regular dreams are dreams in which you relive situations that you experienced the day before again and again. If you have not resolved some kind of earlier conversation within yourself, it can reappear constantly. You might have the same conversation with somebody but in a different, positive way. You can also return to your childhood or any other part of your life that is tied to some event or feeling that has influenced your beliefs and behavior in the current phase of your life. This includes dreams that are linked with your hidden and overt wishes, needs, and desires.

True dreams are the dreams of individuals who are free of all frustrations and problems. These are purely positive dreams.

Divine dreaming is a state in which there are no dreams, no thoughts, where everything both is and is not.

Bioenergy

Bioenergy is an energy that is a key component of the body, and the body can have it in smaller or larger amounts. This is your healing energy that helps you solve your physical problems if you allow it to through your attitude and behavior. If you feed off the negative energies of your emotions and frustrations, you will have little bioenergy. If you nourish yourself with healthy emotions and love, you will have lots of energy and people happily spend time in your company.

There are people who feed off unhealthy energies, for example smoking; which destroys the tissues of your physical body. Often, when you fall and have an open wound, doctors cannot, despite their best efforts, save your hip or hand or foot because your organism's flesh has rotted due to many years of smoking. This shows that you are not living, merely existing.

People who share their bioenergy while healing somebody have to keep in mind that everyone has their own frequency and that those people who have a relatively compatible energy to theirs can be helped to an extent, but they cannot heal them fully.

In addition, such individuals take on the risk that they will retain the energy of the patient in their own energy field. The next risk is that they will be so exhausted by giving their energy that they can fall ill.

After every treatment, the bioenergy therapist must cleanse their energy and rest physically in order to restore their energy.

It is better to look after your bioenergy and nourish it with positive thoughts so that you do not need to put yourself in the situation where you need to ask for help from someone to whom you can cause harm.

Teleportation

Teleportation is the moving of the body to other regions or places. This means that the individual disappears from one place and appears in another.

The process consists of powerful, deep concentration. You lift your material body up to a higher vibrational level using your thoughts, high enough for that from the material body to transform into a pure body of energy. After that, with a clear consciousness, you move and appear in the place where you wish to be, but the process is inverted. Given that every cell in the body has its own intelligence and knows what kind and which function it is responsible for and what its purpose is, an absolutely identical material body is produced to the original one by materializing out of energy and into a material body.

Bilocation

Bilocation is the presence of the material body in two or more locations, or places, at the same time. The process is similar to teleportation except that the energy is divided and forms more new material bodies out of the pure energy of consciousness exactly the same as with teleportation, only with more individuals. It is difficult to maintain several material bodies in various locations because your body's energy searches for reunification. The opposite process, the process of reunifying all the bilocated bodies into a single one, is for many extremely painful. All bodies function independently within a single consciousness because it is the energy of one body, one being.

Telekinesis

Telekinesis is the moving, bending, relocating, and throwing of non-living things with your mind. Via telekinesis, books can be moved, metal objects bent, lights switched off – everything that can be done with the hand – except that the power of thought is much more powerful than physical strength.

Using telekinesis, people lift cars or large vehicles from off their loved ones because willpower acts on their consciousness, which is all-powerful, and when you call on it, it will do everything to help you.

Levitation

Levitation is the ability to be in a weightless state.

One type of levitation is to bring your material body into a state in which gravity does not affect it using the power of your thoughts, and your body can thus freely move in the space above the earth. The body can be up to four meters high in the air, given that a loss in concentration immediately leads to gravity once more beginning to work and your body falls to the ground. People are not permitted a greater height because they might otherwise sustain worse injuries when they fall.

The other type of levitation is affecting objects and non-living things with the power of thought. The larger the object, the better it is to have more people joining in the concentration for levitation. In this way, a more powerful energy is achieved, which leads to the force of gravity no longer affecting that object or non-living thing. As soon as one link is broken, that is, as soon as the concentration of one person in the group decreases or disappears, the non-living thing once again has its gravitational pull. Such powers were frequently used in Ancient Egypt.

Part III
What You Were Given When You Arrived on the Earth

Angels

Angels are highly developed beings that live at a higher frequency than humans and are therefore invisible to the human eye. They are given to humans to help in various situations. There are many more angels than there are humans. As soon as they are born, each individual is assigned an angel that follows them up until they leave the physical world. Angels are sexless beings. They are of various sizes, from the smallest that are just a few centimeters long to those several kilometers long.

Even the smallest angel is physically stronger than the strongest person that walks the Earth.

They are all immeasurably positive and whenever you need them and call on them, they will rush to your aid. There are many kinds of duties that angels perform for humans, in the sense of care and love. Angels' duties are in keeping with their size and power. There are Healing Angels, Helper Angels for various situations, from the all-but-harmless like the possibility of falling or the possibility of some kind of more dangerous accident to Guardian Angels, Angels of the Sacrament, Angel-Doctors, Angels of Love, Earthly Angels, Practical Angels, Angels of Nature Preservation, Angels of Peace and many others.

Angels are stronger than your doubts and fears.

Angels bring light to even the hardest tasks and darkest situations.

If you ask them for protection, angels will most probably help you avoid an accident or misadventure while you are distracted, melancholy, or anxious. Many people are aware of this, but they don't put two and two together because angels can appear in innumerable various shapes and take on the appearance of people so that the person they are helping will experience as little trauma as possible, and not be frightened. Help frequently comes to you in such a form that you all but do not notice it, given that angels are extremely careful and gentle beings that wish to help you (although they do not wish to infringe on the situations and events that happen to you in your life because they know that you have to learn something from these situations).

If you are trusting and ask for help from the angels, it does not matter if you are alone or in a group. They will help you, and you simultaneously help the group because by asking for help, you believe. In so doing, you make it clear that you support love and the people around you are all automatically protected. For example, with your intuition, you can sense a coming danger. You are in a car (alone or with someone) and feel that an accident might occur. You relax and ask an angel to protect you with white light white energy. An accident will probably happen, but you and the people who are with you in the car, given that you are protected, will probably survive it without any consequences.

You only need to ask them for help, and they will always be there for you and alongside you.

If every person were aware of how much help they receive from the spiritual world – and one of the immeasurably large parts are from angels – they would not feel alone and vulnerable. The majority of mothers smother their children with the low energy of worry rather than believing and entrusting their children to their guardian angels. Babies and small children frequently sense and see the presence of their angel, and they frequently play with them too. The more you believe, the more you child will be protected.

You can also turn to your guardian angel when taking care of household tasks. You will notice that it is much easier for you to vacuum or clean the bathroom than it was before. If you are carrying heavy shopping bags, ask him to help you, and you will feel that the bags are lighter. You only have to believe in that which exists.

In the same way, if you find yourself in a situation where you require warmth, you can ask him for help and you will feel, alongside security, immense warmth that will protect you until help arrives.

The function of the Angels of the Sacrament is to give positive energy irrespective of whether the situation is a happy or a sad one for the person. They usually appear in groups. They help people to accept more easily a particular situation and rejoice when they see a positive response. They appear at baptisms to celebrate the soul that has been reincarnated, at weddings to celebrate the union of two people, at divorces to help ease the situation between the former partners, at funerals to await and accompany the soul where it needs to go, at birthday parties, and at all kinds of celebrations.

Angel-Doctors heal using colors given that colors have particular frequencies and are also a part of every body. Every energy center has its color. With these colors, angels clear out the negative energy from the energy field of the individual and align it with the clean colors in order to heal the body of the person that has asked them for this.

Angels of Love work on healing your deep scars that are connected to love. These are jealousy, envy, hatred, anger, and fury towards people that are caused by the insufficient care and understanding that you felt or feel on your side.

Earthly Angels appear in human form, and after fulfilling their purpose, disappear. If a person needs help and cannot manage – but given the distant situation and their future life it is important that they succeed in something – an angel in human form appears, helps them, and then disappears. Only the person whom he has helped can see and sees him. For example, an older woman is asking for help in a railway station, but nobody approaches her. She needs to make a train in order to later catch a plane, and this is very important for her future development. A person appears out of nowhere, shows her the direction, leads her to the train, and seats her. The older woman arrives in time to catch her plane. Or an accident occurs. The person needs to survive, but the ambulance cannot come in time because of certain circumstances and the person at the site of the accident does not known how to help the victims. A person appears out of nowhere, places a hand on the body of the victim, and they begin to breathe. The person then disappears. The ambulance later appears and takes care of the victim, who would not have survived if the angel had not appeared.

Practical Angels help in small situations. For example, you are going to the city during peak hour and you need a parking spot. Before you begin and while you are driving, you ask an angel to create an empty space for you because you are in a hurry, and it is important for you to take care of everything quickly. He will put all his best efforts into making this happen and will lead you to that spot. Listen to your intuition. Or you can ask the angel to look after your car if you find yourself in some unsafe area, and he will do so.

Angels of Nature Preservation manipulate the elements that take care of nature. These are the elements earth, air, fire, and water. When people respect the natural world, they help the angels and, in keeping with the spiritual laws, in return receive help.

Healing Angels help during deeper cleanses of the organism of your frustrations and emotions, where that process have led you into an unwanted physical state.

A Meditation to Connect with Your Guardian Angel:

- Position yourself comfortably in a seated position and relax. You can put on gentle, soothing music, if you like.
- Take a few breaths to relax your material body.
- Call on your guardian angel to come closer to you. Feel how his gentle wings are embracing you and relax in the security. You will probably feel gentle warmth.
- Surrounded by love and with the feeling of safety you have received from your guardian angel, become aware of how much love he is giving you.

- Breathe and absorb all this love. Remind yourself that you deserve to be loved.
- When you are ready, slowly open your eyes and keep that feeling inside of you for a long time.

Reincarnation

Reincarnation is the appearance of a soul in several lives on Earth in order to fulfill its purpose. The Earth is a planet that God created along with the principle of cause and effect. He gave man free will, but He also limited man's knowledge of man's purpose at the moment of birth. It is for this reason that man is pulled into the wheel of his own destiny. Until he fulfils his purpose on Earth, which is a life lived in the truth that we are all one and we are all God because God is an all-pervasive consciousness, the energy of absolute love, man will continue to return to Earth in a physical form.

As God would not leave man in the dark to struggle on his own, He gave man many abilities, such as astral projection and dreams, in which man can understand that he is not merely his physical body but something much more, and something more subtle. In addition, amongst people there are always spiritual individuals who are teachers, who are aware of what man is, and occasionally he sends them His prophets to bring the human race out of the darkness and into the light. Up until now these prophets have been the Buddha (meaning "vigilance"), Muhammed (meaning "peace"), Christ (meaning "light"), Krishna (meaning "light") and Sathya Sai Baba (Sai Baba for short, meaning "father/ mother").

There are three kinds of reincarnation:

- Where a soul reincarnates until it achieves the reason for its existence, which can be between a few and several hundred times
- Where a soul reincarnates only when it needs to in order to help explain the truth and then it consciously and with a goal and purpose reincarnates up to five times but does not enter into a karmic pattern
- Where a soul reincarnates in order to bring light to the Earth, which means "love" and which increases the level of positive energy on Earth and comes to a better understanding of the truth; these are God's Prophets

Part IV
Explanations

Duality

Duality is the same situation examined from two different sides. God created duality so that man could experience his free will.

Duality, as man sees it, consists of two opposing polarities, good and bad. He characterizes it as good when everything goes well for him, when he has a job, money, a partner, and good health. Bad is characterized by the opposite. He connects the good with God's Prophets, the bad with the Devil. Many people believe that God's Prophets exist, but nobody has yet found evidence for the existence of the Devil because he never existed, nor will he ever exist. The Devil is a product of the imagination of humans who had to give a name to negative energy in order to understand the opposite of good.

This is energy with a very low frequency, and a person who has more negative energy therefore has a denser material body. By raising this energy and recognizing the truth and a life lived in love (meaning that he accepts positive energy in himself) man raises his energy. He is lighter. He lives at higher frequencies and in the end reaches nirvana (total blessedness and unity with God).

In Catholicism, when speaking of Adam and Eve, who were thrown out of Paradise (eternal blessedness, eternal truth) because Eve gave Adam an apple from the Tree of Knowledge of Good and Evil and he accepted it, this is not about sin.

Sin in and of itself does not exist. Everything that you do, you do to yourself. The more difficult it is for you to understand who you are, you bring yourself into new events and situations that force you, mainly in the beginning very gently, to realize which path you have to take. If you understand that the aim of your path in life is in goodness and love, you will experience few situations that will need to direct you; instead, you will just listen to your intuition and follow it. Then there are no mistakes or straying; you head directly towards your goal.

Eve represents intuition and consciousness, while Adam represents a logical way of thinking. Intuition encouraged logic in order for God's plan to be realized, which is as it is described in the Book of Genesis: "Be fertile and multiply, fill the earth." Without that first event, there would not be a single person upon the Earth.

This demonstrates that in his life man must first listen to his intuition (the heart, the higher consciousness), and after that, use his logic and he will never do wrong. God created everything as a duality, which in its nature forms a whole, because if it were not this way, man would be separated from everything, even from his very self, never discovering the truth. If you had never known negative energy you would not be able to know its opposite. Moreover, the majority of people know that just by reviving the positive energy of love – your satisfaction, feeling of relaxation, luck, happiness, joy – all the black clouds in your thoughts disappear. After that, you feel better and healthy and fulfilled. This shows you that negative energy really does not exist because you can get rid of it in an instant, while in the opposite situation (which never was the case and never will be because man always longs for the better), you cannot in an instant wipe away the love in your heart, nor the truth. They are steadfast and within you your entire life; you only need to allow them to show themselves to you.

The Symbol of the Cross

The model of the cross shows the structure of man's polarity as a micro-universe. The cross has four directions. When the cross is drawn, every direction has to be at a ninety-degree angle in relation to the other, and they have to be the same length because no one part is any more important than the other.

- The center of the cross represents your heart, your higher consciousness, the center of the Soul
- The left direction represents Eve, your intuition and consciousness, and the right direction Adam, your logic; the perfect balance between yang/yin (the male and female aspects within man),
- The upward direction is good, the downward is bad, and these are the polarities of human experiences as if they were viewed in a mirror because the bad is a mirror image of the good (everything is one; it depends which side you are examining it from).

Every person must understand how they reflect and live these polarities because by balancing the female and male aspects within themselves and understanding that you will be presented with situations that you must view from the good or the bad side because it represents one, you will understand that this is your free will in which manner you will explain a particular event. The more a person is distanced from their center, the more powerfully the polarity that they live is reflected.

In addition to free will, God also gave you the power to choose. Those who understand that they can go no further because they have fallen into a trap (an illusion, uncertainty about life, about their struggle) have a choice. By changing their way of thinking, that light of truth and love in your heart begins to smolder, chasing away all uncertainty, and thus enlightening your being because you are a being of the Light.

Auras

An aura is an energy field that every human being has. The smaller the aura, the more a person feels bad, dissatisfied, frustrated, grumpy, aggressive, and sick. The bigger the aura, the more that person feels calm, good-natured, satisfied, happy, healthy, connected to everybody and everything, and fulfilled.

People who have small aura or damaged (incomplete) aura aim to take energy from others, which mean that they need energy. They do not know how to get it, but a change in mindset and behavior in a positive sense is all that is required. People like this who have pets are usually calmer because pets instinctively sense that their owner needs positive energy and gives it to them selflessly. The majority of pets get sick in this way because they give their owners selfless love, but they do not know how to get rid of the owner's negative energy. They unconsciously receive into their aura, and in this way, they begin developing illnesses.

So be thankful to your pets, cuddle them and take care of them; they are your boundless love that you still need to discover within yourself.

People who have a large aura are extremely positive people. These auras can be up to several kilometers in size. Those people who find themselves in their vicinity, depending on the amount of energy, react in various ways.

Those people who do not have enough energy are always prone to picking fights with everyone and with people with lots of energy because their unconscious physical "I", their ego, learnt to get energy this way. This does not work for them, of course, because positive people never allow themselves to be dragged into something they have already experienced, or they simply know the reason behind this kind of behavior and therefore remain calm. People who have a lot of energy give it unselfishly irrespective of which and what kind of person they find themselves close to, out of sheer love and the understanding that such a person still needs to grow.

Those people who are heading down the path of personal growth enjoy being close to such people and try to connect them. This can lead to conflict, given that people who have a lot of energy cannot be tied to anything or anyone because they alone are free and free from the karmic circle. They understand those people who want to form an attachment and, in the gentlest way possible, they direct them to the right path, the path of liberation.

Kundalini

Kundalini is a band of energy that connects human beings with the Earth and the Universe. There are two centers in the human body through which this band stretches. One is located in the second energy center in the middle of the body, four centimeters below the navel and is responsible for balance in the material body and enables that person to be connected to the earthly, that is, it connects them to the Earth. The second is located in the fourth energy center (the heart) twelve centimeters below the lower line of the neck in the middle of the body, and it is responsible for balance in the spiritual body and allows for connection with the all-knowing, all-encompassing consciousness, the Universe.

The part of the energy band within the body that connects one energy center with the other must be in balance in order to harmonize the energies of the earthly and the spiritual in man.

Collective Consciousness

The collective consciousness is the consciousness of everything living and nonliving on the Earth.

Everything is interconnected and unified. Everything forms one whole.

Your mindset affects not only you and your energy field, but the fields of your household, after that the energy fields of your pets (if you have them), then the energy fields of your plants, the energy fields of your neighbors, the people that you meet every time you go to the store, all the people that you meet at work, that you meet while walking in the city or park, all the plants and animals that you pass by when you walk through the forest, mountains, the ground that you walk on, the good and bad weather; and at the same time, they all, with their various energy fields, affect you.

We know that a person feels bad in the vicinity of someone who needs energy.

We know that a person feels bad in situations where they lose energy on negative and destructive thinking.

We know that a person feels good when they are happily in love.

We know that a person feels good when they live in a harmonious family.

We know that a person feels good while they are walking through a park because the trees give them the positive energy of their boundless love.

We know that a person feels good when it is sunny.

Be careful how you think and the manner in which you express your feelings because everything is connected. The more you think positively, the amount of positive energy in everything around you will automatically increase, and you will thus be blessed with a purification of the body, an increase in your energy, and a life lived in the truth.

Spirits and Souls

The Spirit is a link with God and God himself, consciousness itself, while the Soul is that small part of His consciousness and His boundless love that God gave you so that you could enter a physical body and live this wonderful life.

Many people are afraid to leave their physical body because they have been taught incorrectly. Nowadays, people are taught that they are primarily their physical body and that the soul makes up a part of that body. The opposite is in fact true. In order to feel and grow you have to have a material body, the shape that a soul takes on in order to make this possible.

Fear of leaving one's physical body also leads to the belief that after its physical death the soul goes to heaven or hell. On their own, heaven and hell do not exist, but expressions of heaven and hell exist which appear after physical death based on a person's thoughts and beliefs while in human form.

If, after their physical death, a person is not convinced enough that an angel, one of their deceased relatives, a saint or some other being of light will come for them, the soul will remain for some time in the so-called Grey Zone.

The Grey Zone is a space where souls remain for some time until they understand that it is not what they need. It is the space that they will inhabit after leaving their physical body up until the departure for a higher dimension. People can remain in the Grey Zone for centuries, given that this zone does not have either time or space. These are people who do not wish to give up their own wealth, and so in the Grey Zone they materialize their Earthly kingdom in their minds. In this zone, there are also people who do not understand that they have died and so wander the Earth through familiar places in the hope that someone will notice them, but this does not happen.

These two situations are the most common. In the first case, they realize sooner or later that it is time for them to move on, and a being of light whose duty it is to lead them appears in the very same moment and leads them away. In the second case, apparitions of souls that have not yet left their former Earthly home have been known to appear or the moving of objects and things can occur when someone's soul becomes restless. A soul becomes restless when it realizes that it no longer has its physical form and that it is in a different dimension. If you cannot go to a church institution and pray a requiem, all you need to do is light a candle at home and carefully pray for the soul to be shown its path. Someone will appear in that same moment and help them. Sometimes a soul may appear to you who need help, but they are not familiar to you from this Earthly life. The approach is the same because you always pray for the soul, not the person.

Many of a departed soul's nearest and dearest do not wish to let them go because they previously had a feeling of safety (for the most part) and they want that to remain the same. In this way, they do not allow the soul to follow its path but instead selfishly push it to forcibly remain on Earth. It then remains in the grey zone until you finally realize that you need to let it go. The soul chooses for itself when it will leave the physical for the spiritual dimension; this is one of the expressions of choice and free will.

There are of course souls who leave the physical for the spiritual, but of their own free will, remain alongside their loved ones because they need to protect them after leaving behind their physical bodies. Then it is on them to decide when they want to leave.

The fact that a soul, after leaving its physical body, can create heaven or hell is but a temporary thing. The path that it has to take, it will take, and sooner or later it will arrive where it is supposed to be.

Heaven and hell are artificial creations, as well as the belief that human beings live only once upon the Earth. This is a fairly restrictive way of thinking that emerged from ignorance and the desire for power. Power usually creates fear, and fear produces obedience. These are all very unhealthy feelings that forcibly tie human beings to the physical.

Spirituality/Spiritual People

Spirituality is your openness to the higher consciousness. If you are an open person, if you listen to your intuition and behave in keeping with the truth, you are a spiritual person. A spiritual person is calm, understanding, modest (they do not stand out or raise themselves above others), peaceful, serene, and has all of the calming characteristics. Such a person will help you in a correct way, which will very frequently be different from what you had thought would be good for you. Sometimes they will simply turn their backs on you, and you will not know why. The reason for this is that you are not yet ready, or you have to understand their approach and, in this way, grow. When you need them, they will appear once again and always when you are at a turning-point or when you need help taking a positive step in your life.

Spiritual Development in Relation to Astral Projection and Sex

The majority of so-called spiritual teachers tell all their students that, if they wish to develop in the spiritual sense and if they wish to succeed at astral projection, they have to abstain from sex. This is the truth only when sex is had merely for the satisfying of the body's needs. (Sex should be had only to strengthen the connection between two people. This leads to the increasing of positive energy in the body and the development of a better relationship and strengthening of understanding between partners.)

Healthy sex leads to a harmonizing of your material body and along with your spiritualization leads to the harmonization of the entire body.

Another incorrectly taught idea is that during spiritualization you can eat everything but only in small amounts. If you wish to become spiritualized, understand the truth, and live in love, it is necessary to willingly abstain from everything that you know does harm to your body because it decreases your energy and your body becomes denser and thus darker. Spiritual people have light bodies.

Astral projection does not depend on whether you eat meat or something that is bad for your body or if you have sex or not. It is given to you at birth. If you wish to once again call on that memory, practice, but before going to sleep, eat very little or nothing in order for your unconscious to be directed towards your wish and not on the difficult digestion of food.

Teachers/Gurus

This is a person who has travelled the entire path of knowledge and who can help in finding, explaining, and understanding the truth. There are very few people like this on Earth, so be careful that, because of your desire for enlightenment, you do not come across a person who cannot offer you what you are searching for and need. People who call themselves teachers/gurus today are, for the most part, people who have headed down the path of their own spiritualization at full speed or are people who enjoy being the center of attention in order to satisfy their ego. The first group of people can help to a certain extent; for the most part, they have not understood the true meaning of the truth, but they are on the right path towards realizing their goal. Some of them learned from Eastern teachers, but keep in mind that those teachers, too, were once students and that every teacher has a different understanding of the same things. Only the highest-ranked lamas from Tibet, Tibetan hermits who live in caves high in the mountains of Tibet, Zen Buddhist priests who live completely apart from civilization, and some very enlightened people who live all around the world can truly help on that journey – only if you are looking for a teacher in human form.

Anybody can head down this path, and alone it is important that one decides, gives oneself over to one's intuition, and believes because then you will be sent people from whom you will be able to learn something. You will be sent books and events, and just by noticing the changes, you will change yourself in a positive sense and step by step you will arrive at the truth.

Healing/Curing Illnesses

The basic difference between healing an illness and curing it is that healing heals and completely frees one from the cause of the illness (the initial mental structure that is the cause of every illness) that a person has. Healing is done on the mental, psychological, and in the end, on the physical body. Curing illnesses is done only on the level of the physical body, treating only the symptom, the illness, and in this way the cause of the illness, the problem, is not resolved. This means that it is highly probable that the illness will reappear in the same or in some other place if you do not change your way of thinking and behaving.

Mental Illnesses

Mental illnesses are illnesses that affect a person's mental body. There are two kinds of people with mental illnesses. In both cases, the energy field of that person is highly distorted and doctors treating them with Western medicine cannot have almost any success.

With the first type, the energy body of the person is so damaged that it contains holes, which do not allow the material body to function normally. Medicines only worsen the already difficult situation in the energy field of such a person.

With the second type, which is more complicated, the person's energy field is all but completely outside of their material body.

Holes in a person's energy field provide good conditions for beings from a second dimension to settle in. These beings are beings that are still developing and so search for the energy field of a higher being because they believe that they will develop more quickly in this way. However, everyone has their own developmental cycle, and so do they. This does not happen when there is an energy field that is whole. The majority of people have such a field.

When they enter into a person's energy field these beings cause, primarily, a feeling of discomfort. The person begins to act strangely, to shriek, to rage, beat themselves and do everything in their power to get rid of their unwanted neighbor/s. The majority of people in this situation search for Catholic priests, exorcists, or those who work on freeing the energy field from beings from second dimension (they call this freeing the soul from demons).

Such beings from second dimension flee from the buildup of positive energy, because in this case, the person's energy field is filled in and forms a proper shape and there is no longer space for them.

You can help such people by praying for them that love fills their entire body and that their energy field is healed and mended. For people whose energy field is all but outside their material body, you can also pray that they receive a full, total, shining energy field full of love that completely envelops their material body.

With God's help and an understanding of the truth, everything is possible; therefore, believe and pray.

Colors

Every color has its own vibration and energy that influences us even when we are not aware of it. Bright red will energize us, while green will balance us out, and blue will calm us down. Yellow helps us with concentration, and the color indigo (blue violet) soothes our thoughts. The colors that we paint our walls with will have an impact on us. We choose to wear colors that express our identity or provide us with something that we lack.

When the appropriate colors are directed in order to heal a body, the energy of every color blends with the cells of the body, energizes them, and thus breaks down the negative energy from the cells. While one illness can respond to one color, another illness will respond to another.

For example, cancer responds to green because this is the color of the center of the heart, and we need the center of the heart to be open and relaxed in order for it to effectively accept the color for healing illness. People in shock or those who need to be calmed down respond to the color indigo. A person with depression will respond well to warm red and orange.

If you do not know which color works best for you when healing with colors, the easiest and best thing to do is use the color white. You have certainly seen in physics class how passing white light through a prism creates a whole spectrum of rainbow colors. These same colors can be found in our bodies. For this reason, feel free to use the color white to heal all illnesses. White is a clean, protective color and the strongest for healing because it reflects light.

Colors also simultaneously show the passivity or activeness of a particular person. For this reason, people should wear colors that make them happy and shine.

You should avoid the color black because it takes away energy. It shows that you are a passive person and that you are not really living. This why black is very much in fashion these days. Black is not essentially a color; it is the absence of color. Black consumes light, consumes energy. This is why people in many nations wear it during periods of mourning. Those who grieve have little energy because energy is tied to pain and deals with it.

Many people today wear black because they are in fact grieving for a loss of love and vibrancy; they exclude colors from their lives, which means that they are grieving because of the loss of a whole spectrum of their emotions.

People who predominantly wear black are people who consume others' energy. Only those who live in ignorance seek contact with people who like black. They do not have the colorful, wide-awake eyes of love. They have a weakened capacity for love, so everything is already "black in their eyes", both within and outside of them.

Black can of course be worn from time to time, but for particular events in order for a person to appear elegant and sophisticated, but only in those cases.

Gray is also one of the colors that are fashionable today. This is a softer shade of black, so try to exchange it for colors that are more cheerful.

Live your life in the colors that God has given you. You are surrounded by colors; use them for your own improvement and happiness.

Exercises

Prayer

Prayer is a very powerful way to raise your energy and make your body healthier and to keep it in this state. Always pray only for yourself in the sense of increasing the love in your energy field. In this way, you have an impact on the health and improvement of all five of your bodies – of your material body. You strengthen it and constantly show it how much you love it, and in return, it showers you with beneficial health and love.

A prayer always has to have a positive focus. Pray wherever you happen to be, whomever you find yourself with; pray always and constantly.

A prayer might look like this:

- Thank you, God, for sending me a friend that understands me and I him so that we can support one another in everything
- Thank you, God, for this beautiful day (even if it is raining outside) – in this way you stop being, as it is called today, a weather sensitive person
- Thank you, God, for the fact that I caught the tram on time to get to work
- Thank you, God, for the breakfast that allows me to normalize my blood pressure (Then your blood pressure will stabilize, and you will not have problems when the weather changes.)
- Thank you, God, for these healthy vegetables that I have prepared for myself (and for my family) because they will give me enough energy

and fill up my body in the way that is best for me (us)

- Thank you, God, for this wonderful woman/man (a wife is someone with whom you are married, a woman is a person who is a part of you; a woman is not the same as a wife, she is much more, the same is true for the difference between a man and a husband) – just by praying you change the energy field around you both and raise it, and your relationship improves as a result
- Thank you, God, for the fact that I managed to make all the connections I needed at work, all the facts, and I quickly found the right solution with Your guidance
- Thank you, God, for this well-made business deal that will make both sides happy and particularly the users on both sides and
- Dear God, I pray that I will settle in perfectly at my new job, that I will have business partners with whom I will get on well and that we will complete one another
- Dear God, please send me a person who is... (list the exact positive characteristics of the desired person)
- Dear God, please give me concentration and intelligence to pass the exam to my greatest satisfaction
- Dear God, please....

When doing this always think about how happy and pleased you are and feel it in your body.

Pray for whatever you like, but the prayer has to be directed towards your own wellbeing first of all, and then to everyone else.

Meditation – A Breathing Exercise

This exercise works to clear your cells of negative energy and at once fills them with positive energy. Proper breathing balances the energy in your whole body so that you can move freely and automatically removes energy blockages and decreases the risk of getting sick.

Find some time every day, if possible before you go to sleep so that you can clear your body of the thoughts that have built up.

You need between ten and twenty minutes for this exercise.

Do every inhale and exhale three, six, nine, twelve times because the number three is related to your unconscious. When once you have done the exercise, your unconscious perceives (realizes) that something has happened. The second time you do the exercise, your unconscious realizes that it should pay attention to it. The third time you repeat the exercise, your unconscious has accepted the new situation.

You must be relaxed and not force yourself to breathe properly at once because many people have learnt to breathe only with their lungs while the rest of the body has been ignored. In general, men breathe more correctly than women do. You should breathe only through your nose. In this way, those that have a problem with their sinuses and airways can fix it and heal.

- Position yourself comfortably in an armchair or on a chair. It is important that your back is straight, in order for your kundalini to be straight and for your entire body to balance and heal. If you are sick, stiff, or if it is difficult for you to sit and because of this you cannot straighten your back, God will understand. Dedicate the exercise to him and believe. Ask him to help your back and spine heal.
- Ask your higher consciousness for guidance.

You inhale by first slowly (in the beginning however works best for you) filling your lungs with air, then your diaphragm (the region between the lungs and the belly) and in the end the abdomen (the lower part of the belly).

- With every breath you breathe in white energy that permeates and heals all the cells in your body.

Stop breathing for a moment. Beginners should keep breathing, until through practice they reach a level where their body reacts positively to the possibility of stopping their breath.

Exhaling is the opposite; you slowly press the air from your abdomen, then your diaphragm, and in the end from your lungs.

- With every exhale you breathe out black energy from your body which is made up of negative feelings and thoughts that have built up from every one of your cells.

Stop breathing for a moment. Beginners should keep breathing until through practice they reach a level where their body reacts positively to the possibility of stopping their breath.

Repeat the exercise.

An Exercise for Loosening the Neck

You should stretch only until you feel comfortable.

This exercise works to loosen and stretch the muscles in the neck and back, which also relieves tension in the shoulders.

It gets rid of pain and takes pressure off the neck vertebrae.

It increases circulation towards the brain.

It relaxes and calms.

It decreases high blood pressure.
You need between ten and twenty minutes for this exercise. Do every inhale and exhale three, six, nine, twelve times. Try to relax as much as you can.

- Position yourself comfortably in an armchair or on a chair; it is important that your back is straight.
- Inhale, the head is still and looks forwards.

- While exhaling, turn your head to one side and hold your breath a little.
- While inhaling, bring your head back to its original position with eyes looking forwards and hold your breath a little.
- With the next exhale, turn your head to the other side and hold your breath a little.
- With your next inhale, bring your head back to its original position and hold your breath a little.

You can do the same exercise by tipping your head gently and slowly backwards as far as it goes, do not overdo it) when breathing in and forwards to your chest (as far as it does, do not overdo it) when breathing out.

You can also do this exercise by making circles with your head. Begin with your head gently and slowly tipped towards one shoulder. When inhaling, the circular part goes backwards to the other shoulder, and when breathing out make a circle towards the front and the first shoulder. In this way, one breath in and one breath out make up the entire circle.

Repeat the exercise.

The Double Triangle Exercise

You should stretch only until you feel comfortable.

This exercise works to stretch, strengthen, and activate the muscles of the spine.

It activates the circulation in the muscles of the shoulders and arms.

It eliminates tension, nerves and insomnia.

You need between ten and twenty minutes for this exercise. Do every inhale and exhale three, six, nine, twelve times. Try to relax as much as you can.

- Stand with your feet together. Lower your arms by your sides so that your palms are turned towards your body. Stretch your fingers towards the floor.
- When inhaling, join your palms behind your back and lean backwards as far as is comfortable for you; hold your breath a little.
- When exhaling, lean forwards at a 135-degree angle to the floor at most, and stretch your hands with your palms together on your back towards the ceiling as much as you can (your back must be straight), hold your breath a little.
- When breathing in, stand up straight and hold your breath as much as is comfortable.
- When breathing out, bring your hands back into the position from the first step.

Repeat the exercise.

The Statue Exercise

You should stretch only until you feel comfortable.

This exercise works to strengthen the pelvic muscles.

It prevents problems with the lumbar part of the spine.

It improves concentration.

It relaxes and calms.

It lowers high blood pressure.

You need between ten and twenty minutes for this exercise. Do every inhale and exhale three, six, nine, twelve times. Try to relax as much as you can.

- Crouch down and sit on your heels, your hands are relaxed in your lap (do not cross either your hands or your legs); your head should be held up.
- Lift yourself into a crouching position and step out with your left leg so that your body is in line with the leg that remains in a crouching position and place both palms on your left knee
- When breathing in, spread your hands to the side and stretch them out horizontally at the height of your shoulder.
- When breathing out, bend your body to the side and back and left, then with your left hand touch your right heel while your right palm remains on your left knee. Hold your breath a little. Look backwards.
- When breathing in, straighten your body and spread your arms at shoulder height and hold your breath for a little.
- When breathing out, lower both palms to your left knee.

Repeat the whole exercise in the opposite direction with your right leg.

The Sun Salutation Exercise

You should stretch only until you feel comfortable.
It works to strengthen the muscles in your arms and shoulders.

It strengthens the back muscles and decreases back pains.

It develops your sense of balance.

You need between ten and twenty minutes for this exercise. Do every inhale and exhale three, six, nine, twelve times. Try to relax as much as you can.

- Crouch down and sit on your heels; your hands are relaxed in your lap (do not cross either your hands or your legs); your head should be held up
- Lift yourself into a crouching position and step out with your right leg as far as you can (the left leg is in an all but horizontal position in relation to the floor and the body almost upright).
- When breathing in, lift your arms above your head and join your palms, bend the upper part of your body so that it is all but vertical on the floor, and lift your head; press your hips gently towards the front.
- Take a few breaths in and out in this position.
- When breathing out, first return to a crouching position, and then into the next position.

Repeat the exercise in the opposite direction with your left leg.

To live Love, to live in Love and to give Love, that is why we are here, to be in Love with ourselves, with everyone and everything!

You are all of these things, so use them! Be what you are, God's child of light!

Biography

A continuous search for the truth is the driving force behind the life and work of Renata Francetić. She lives in Zagreb, Croatia, Europe.

From a very young age, she began examining human behavior in various situations. After the age of twenty, she began her research into human psychology, medicine, sociology, behaviorism, and mysticism. In her early thirties, she began studying healing using natural remedies, energies, proper nutrition, and their connection with exercise and a proper diet. She began dealing with metaphysics, quantum physics and the correlation and connections between human energiesand nature in her late thirties. She studies the meaning of angels and the dogmas of thelargest religious groups in the world. She also studiesthe significance of plants, animals and changes in nature with respect to the conscious and unconscious actions of people, as well as the reasons for large and aggressive changes over the past twenty years in the behavior of Mother Earth as the nurturer of everything that is connected to her. Over the past few years, she has begun studying the meaning and influence of ancient cultures and their impact on the growth and development of civilization. The techniques she uses in her daily life are meditation, healing, self-help, a proper diet, and an organized and disciplined lifestyle.

Thanks to her inexhaustible curiosity, she is constantly presented with new fields of study, one of them being hypnotherapy. In her rich life, and owing to her knowledge and experience, she has helped many people with advice and therapy. She has concluded, through her considerable experience in working with people and studying their behavior, that all people are primarily unhappy and displeased with their lives because they long for love and search for it outside of themselves, instead of within. Because everything starts from within a person towards somebody or something, the path is never the reverse. The reason why a large number of people do not tell the truth, are arrogant, quarrel, curse, and are depressed is their separation from God.

Her lifestyle, her positive energy, and immense generosity inspires people around her to make changes in themselves and live fuller and happier lives.

Renata Francetić is also the author of the book *The Power of the Truth*.

Made in the USA
Las Vegas, NV
14 September 2022

55297789R00142